AF520902

Dr. Singh's

NEET PG MCQ's

for Dental Students

ANATOMY Question Bank

Based on Standard Textbooks

Dr. Brijendra Singh
MBBS, MS, DNB, MNAMS
Additional Professor
Department of Anatomy
All Indian Institute of Medical Sciences (AIIMS)
Jodhpur - 342 005 (India)

SCIENTIFIC
PUBLISHERS

Published by
SCIENTIFIC PUBLISHERS (INDIA)

Jodhpur –

5 A, New Pali Road
P.O. Box 91
Jodhpur - 342 001 INDIA

Delhi –

4806/24, Ansari Road
Daryaganj
New Delhi - 110 002 INDIA

ISBN:

Visit the Scientific Publishers (India) website at
http://www.scientificpub.com

Printed in India

Dedicated to

My children

Vyomika Singh & Kostubh Singh

for helping me in preparing and editing this book

my wife

Dr. Ritu Singh

for positive suggestions, ideas and continuous encouragement

My parent college

Teachers, Students & Staff of MLB Medical College, Jhansi

My students past & present

for appreciating my way of teaching - ABC of life that is - Aim, Basics & Competition and expecting more simpler & interesting way of Anatomy teaching from my side.

My friends & well wishers

from

All India Institute of Medical Sciences (AIIMS), Jodhpur, India

PREFACE

First of all I am thankful to all of my students present and past who kept me reminding continuously about the need of small, simple, handy and really concise book of anatomy subject as per their new syllabus and as per latest guidelines of **Dental Council of India. Now-a-days the best exams are supposed to be those which are having Multiple Choice Questions ie MCQ's as integral part** because of two important reasons, First easy to conduct and uniform evaluation for all students, that is no bias, Second **MCQ's** checks memory/recall memory/ reasoning & ability to be precise in terms of reading/understanding and speed with ability to record answers with accuracy too. **"Dr. Singh's NEET PG MCQ's for Dental Students"** is helpful as a complete Question Bank for **fast revision during examination** and will certainly help them to secure full marks in **Postgraduate Entrance Examinations**. One shall remember that **MCQ's** are **the only questions which are asked in PG Entrance Examinations.** Keeping all this in mind and realizing the need of this type of systematic and authentic book on subject as well as continuous demand from various groups of students, this **MCQ** book **"Dr. Singh's NEET PG MCQ's for Dental Students"** is crafted for you all, to make your dreams of getting **PG of your choice** through **NEET PG Entrance Exam.**

All the best for your future ventures......

Good luck & Happy reading .....

Dr. Brijendra Singh
MBBS, MS, DNB, MNAMS
Additional Professor of Anatomy
AIIMS Jodhpur India
E-mail: drbrijendrasingh@gmail.com

ACKNOWLEDGEMENT

First of all my sincere thanks to **Prof. Sanjeev Misra CEO & Director of AIIMS, Jodhpur, India,** for his inspiration, unconditional support & continuous encouragement to create & complete my book **"Dr. Singh's NEET PG MCQ's for Dental Students"**. I am also thankful to my colleagues from department of Anatomy at AIIMS, Jodhpur for their continuous and positive attitude for making this book better and student friendly.

I am also thankful to my childrens Vyomika Singh & Kostubh Singh for helping me in this book and wife Dr. Ritu Singh, for positive suggestions, ideas and continuous encouragement. I am thankful to my students past & present for appreciating my way of teaching - ABC of life that is - Aim, Basics & Competition and expecting more simpler & interesting way of Anatomy teaching from my side I am thankful to my friends & well wishers from All India Institute of Medical Sciences (AIIMS), Jodhpur, India

I am very much thankful to Mr. Tanay Sharma, Managing Director, Scientific Publishers (India), Jodhpur for timely workup editing and final printing.

I am and will remain indebted to almighty **God Lord Krishna** with folded hands for his blessings so that my book **"Dr. Singh's NEET PG MCQ's for Dental Students"** could become a reality and will be useful for readers today, tomorrow & ever.

Thanks & All the best....

Dr. Brijendra Singh
Additional Professor of Anatomy
AIIMS Jodhpur India

CONTENTS

Section - 3
Embryology

Section - 4
Histology

Section - 1
Head & Neck

Chapter 1

Osteology of Head & Neck

1. Hyoid bone in the neck corresponds to–
(A) C2 vertebra
(B) C3 vertebra
(C) C4 vertebra
(D) C5 vertebra

2. Cricoid cartilage in the neck corresponds to –
(A) C5
(B) C5-C6
(C) C6
(D) C7

3. Upper border and notch of thyroid cartilage corresponds to-
(A) C2-C3
(B) C3-C4
(C) C4-C5
(D) C5-C6

4. Thyroid cartilage in the neck corresponds to –
(A) C2-C3
(B) C3-C4
(C) C4-C5
(D) C5-C6

5. Most projecting part of face is-
(A) chin
(B) nose
(C) eyes
(D) zygomas

6. Skull is made up of
(A) 20 bones
(B) 21 bones
(C) 22 bones
(D) 23 bones

7. Paired bones in cranium are-
(A) parietal
(B) temporal
(C) parietal & temporal
(D) parietal, temporal & zygomas

8. Unpaired bones in cranium is/are-
(A) frontal
(B) occipital
(C) ethmoid
(D) all of the above

9. Unpaired bones in the cranium is -
(A) ethmoid
(B) sphenoid
(C) occipital
(D) all of the above

10. True statement is-
(A) cranium is made up of 14 bones
(B) cranium is made up of 22 bones
(C) cranium is made up of 8 bones
(D) cranium is made up of 4 paired & 4 unpaired bones

11. Facial skelton consists of –
(A) 12 bones
(B) 14 bones
(C) 8 bones
(D) 22 bones

12. All are unpaired bones except-
(A) frontal
(B) occipital
(C) inferior nasal concha
(D) vomer

13. Structures passing through - petro-tympanic fissure are-
(A) chorda- tympani nerve
(B) anterior ligament of malleus
(C) both of the above
(D) none of the above

14. Structures passing through - petro-tympanic fissure are-
(A) chorda- tympani nerve
(B) anterior ligament of malleus
(C) anterior tympanic artery
(D) all of the above

15. All are true about lateral incisive foramina-
(A) two in number present in lateral wall of incisive fossa
(B) leads to nasal cavity through incisive canal
(C) greater palatine vessels & nasopalatine nerve pass through
(D) all of the above

16. All are true about median incisive foramina-
(A) two in number present anterior & posterior wall of incisive fossa
(B) left nasopalatine nerve passes through anterior foramen
(C) right nasopalatine nerve passes through posterior foramen
(D) all of the above

17. All are true about palate-vaginal canal except-
(A) b/w sphenoidal process of palatine & root of medial pterygoid plate
(B) pharyngeal nerve a branch from pterygo-palatine ganglion passes through it
(C) pharyngeal artery-a branch from third part of maxillary artery passes through it
(D) all of the above

18. All are true about pterygoid canal except-
(A) connects posterior wall of fora-men lacerum to pterygopalatine fossa
(B) connects anterior wall of foramen lacerum to pterygopalatine fossa
(C) Vidian nerve passes through it
(D) vessels of pterygoid canal

19. True about carotid canal is-
(A) located on inferior surface of petrous temporal bone
(B) internal carotid artery with sympathetic plexus around it
(C) emissary vein connecting pharyngeal venous plexus to cavernous venous sinus
(D) all of the above

20. True about tympanic canaliculus is-
(A) chordatympani nerve
(B) auricular branch of vagus nerve
(C) tympanic branch of glossopharyngeal nerve
(D) none of the above

21. True about mastoid canaliculus is-
(A) chordatympani nerve
(B) auricular branch of vagus nerve
(C) tympanic branch of glossopharyngeal nerve
(D) none of the above

22. All are true about Arnold's nerve except-
(A) present in lateral wall of jugular fossa
(B) alderman's nerve or arnold's nerve is present
(C) auricular branch of glossopharyngeal nerve
(D) auricular branch of vagus nerve

23. All are true about stylomastoid foramen except-
(A) facial nerve
(B) stylomastoid artery branch of occipital artery
(C) stylomastoid artery branch of posterior auricular artery
(D) facial nerve exits and enters into parotid gland

24. Largest and strongest bone of the face is-
(A) maxilla
(B) zygomatoc bone
(C) mandible
(D) inferior nasal concha

25. Mandibular foramen provides passage to-
(A) inferior alveolar nerve
(B) inferior alveolar artery
(C) inferior alveolar vein
(D) all of the above

26. Angle of mandible is in children-
(A) 110^0
(B) 120^0
(C) 130^0
(D) 140^0

27. Angle of mandible is in adults-
(A) 110^0
(B) 120^0
(C) 130^0
(D) 140^0

28. Angle of mandible is in old-
(A) 110^0
(B) 120^0
(C) 130^0
(D) 140^0

29. Mandibular canal
(A) runs near the lower border in old age
(B) runs near the upper border in old age
(C) runs near the upper border in children
(D) runs near the lower border in children and old both

30. True about the position of mental foramen is-
(A) present close to lower border in children
(B) present midway in adults
(C) present close to upper border in old age
(D) all are true

31. In adults-
(A) coronoid process is above the condyloid process
(B) coronoid process is below the condyloid process
(C) coronoid process is equal the condyloid process
(D) none of the above

32. All are true about the mandible of children –
(A) mental foramen closer to lower border
(B) angle of mandible is 140^0
(C) coronoid process is above the condyloid process
(D) all of the above

33. All are true about the mandible of old–
(A) mental foramen closer to upper border
(B) angle of mandible is 140^0
(C) coronoid process is above the condyloid process
(D) all of the above

34. All are true about the mandible of adults except –
(A) mental foramen closer to upper border
(B) angle of mandible is 110^0
(C) coronoid process is below the condyloid process
(D) mandibular canal runs parallel to mylohyoid line

35. In females true about mandible is-
(A) smaller and thinner
(B) height of body is lesser
(C) angle of mandible is inverted
(D) all of the above

36. In males true about mandible is-
(A) larger and thicker
(B) height of body is more
(C) angle of mandible is everted
(D) all of the above

37. In males true about mandible is-
(A) inferior border of mandible is irregular
(B) chin is quadrilateral
(C) angle of mandible is everted
(D) all of the above

38. In females true about mandible is-
(A) inferior border of mandible is smooth
(B) chin is rounded
(C) angle of mandible is inverted
(D) all of the above

39. Mandible is ossified in
(A) membrane
(B) cartilage
(C) both
(D) none

40. True about ossification of mandible is-
(A) area around mandibular canal ossifies in membrane
(B) area proximal to mandibular foramen and area distal to mental foramen ossifies in cartilage
(C) it ossifies in meckel's cartilage
(D) all are true

41. All are true for mandible except-
(A) second bone to ossify
(B) bone derived from 1st branchial arch
(C) at symphysis menti bony union starts from below upwards in first year of life
(D) all are true

42. All are true for maxilla-
(A) body contains air sinus
(B) orbital surface has canal for infraorbital nerve & vessels
(C) infratemporal surface has foramina for posterior superior vessels & nerves
(D) all of the above

43. At birth following are of adult size
(A) tympanic cavity
(B) tympanic membrane
(C) ear ossicles
(D) all of the above

44. True about zygomatic bone is-
(A) ossify in membrane
(B) horizontal fissure sometimes divides into upper & lower half
(C) this feature is seen in Mongolian races called OS Japonicum
(D) all of the above

45. All are parts of ethmoid bone except-
(A) cribriform plate
(B) crista galli
(C) inferior nasal concha
(D) superior nasal concha

46. True about cervical vertebra is all except-
(A) foramen transversarium is typical feature
(B) C3 to C6 are typical cervical vertebra
(C) antero posterior diameter is greater than Transverse diameter
(D) cervical vertebrae are seven in number

47. Joints of luschka-Unco-vertebral joints are seen in
(A) thoracic vertebra
(B) cervical vertebra
(C) lumbar vertebra
(D) sacrum

48. True about cervical vertebre is all except-
(A) vertebral foramen is triangular & larger than body
(B) spine is straight & bifid
(C) lateral margins of the body shows projections laterally
(D) all of the above

49. First cervical vertebrae is –
(A) atypical
(B) no body & no spine
(C) called atlas
(D) all of the above

50. Lingual artery forms loop around the
(A) above the body of hyoid bone
(B) above the greater cornu of hyoid bone
(C) above the lesser cornu of hyoid bone
(D) below the body of hyoid bone

51. Superior surface of posterior arch of atlas is related to-
(A) vertebral artery
(B) 1st cervical nerve
(C) vertebral artery & 1st cervical nerve
(D) none of the above

52. Features of 1st cervical vertebra are-
(A) absence of body & spine
(B) superior articular facets are concave and elongated
(C) long transverse process
(D) all of the above

53. True about 2nd cervical vertebra is-
(A) presence of odontoid process
(B) small transverse process without anterior tubercle
(C) bifid spine
(D) all of the above

54. Vertebral artery does not pass through foramen transversarium of-
(A) C6
(B) C7
(C) C1
(D) none of the above

55. True about C7 vertebra is-
(A) spine is long & bifid
(B) spine is short stout and bifid
(C) spine is long & non-bifid
(D) none of the above

56. Most commonly fractured cranial fossa is-
(A) anterior cranial fossa
(B) middle cranial fossa
(C) posterior cranial fossa
(D) all of the above

57. Largest fontanelle is-
(A) anterior fontanelle
(B) lateral fontanelle
(C) posterior fontanellea
(D) all of the above

58. Most fragile bone in of skull is-
(A) sphenoid
(B) ethmoid
(C) squamous part of temporal
(D) maxilla

59. Metopic suture is present in-
(A) parietal
(B) frontal
(C) occipital
(D) temporal

60. Crista gali is a part of-
(A) hyoid
(B) ethmoid
(C) sphenoid
(D) frontal

61. Sutural junction between frontal & parietal bone is called
(A) nasion
(B) inion
(C) bregma
(D) lambda

62. All are necessary for tooth formation except-
(A) vestibular lamina
(B) dental lamina
(C) membrana preformativa
(D) dental papilla

63. Mandible is formed by-
(A) meckles cartilage
(B) enchondral ossification
(C) intramembranous ossification
(D) B+C

64. Two halves of mandible unite at symphysis menti at-
(A) 10th week of intrauterine life
(B) 7th month of intrauterine life
(C) first year of life
(D) at puberty

65. Gomphosis is a term used for-
(A) gingival attachment
(B) degenerative disease of gums
(C) tooth root attachment to alveolar sockets
(D) TM-Joint

66. Lingula is the process seen on-
(A) in posterior 2/3 of the tongue
(B) on outer aspect of mastoid process
(C) ramus of mandible on external surface
(D) ramus of mandible on interrnal surface

67. Sagittal suture is suture present between-
(A) parietal & frontal bones
(B) parietal & temporal bones
(C) parietal & parietal bones
(D) parietal & occipital bones

68. Meniscus of Temporomandibular joint is made up of-
(A) fibrocartilage
(B) fibrous tissue
(C) articular cartilage
(D) none of the above

69. Meniscus of Temporomandibular joint in elderly is made up of-
(A) fibrocartilage
(B) fibrous tissue
(C) articular cartilage
(D) none of the above

70. Pterygoid plates are part of-
(A) inner aspect of ramus of mandible
(B) temporal bone
(C) sphenoid bone
(D) maxilla

71. Structure passing through foramen rotundum is-
(A) mandibular nerve
(B) opthalmic nerve
(C) maxillary nerve
(D) trigeminal nerve

72. Widest cervical vertebra-
(A) C1
(B) C2
(C) C6
(D) C7

73. Cervical vertebra with thickest spinous process-
(A) C1
(B) C2
(C) C5
(D) C7

74. Hangman fracture is fracture of –
(A) pedicle of C1
(B) pedicle of C2
(C) pedicle of C3
(D) pedicle of C7

Answersheet

1. B, 2. C, 3. B, 4. C, 5. B, 6. C, 7. C, 8. D, 9. D, 10. C, 11. B, 12. C, 13. C, 14. D, 15. D, 16. D, 17. D, 18. A, 19. D, 20. C, 21. B, 22. C, 23. B, 24. C, 25.D, 26. D, 27. A, 28. D, 29. B, 30. D, 31. B, 32. D, 33. D, 34. A, 35. D, 36. D, 37. D, 38. D, 39. C, 40.D, 41. D, 42. D, 43. D, 44. D, 45. C, 46. C, 47. B, 48. D, 49. D, 50. B, 51. C, 52. D, 53. D, 54. B, 55. C, 56. B, 57. A, 58. B, 59. B, 60. B, 61. C, 62. A, 63. D, 64. C, 65. C, 66. D, 67. C, 68. B, 69. A, 70. C, 71. C, 72. A, 73. B, 74. B

Chapter 2

Scalp Face & Temple

1. Scalp is made up of-
   (A) three layers
   (B) four layers
   (C) five layers
   (D) six layers

2. Scalp is commonest site for-
   (A) sebaceous cysts
   (B) berry eneurysms
   (C) both
   (D) none

3. Epicranial aponeurosis is-
   (A) formed by occipitofrontalis muscle & corresponds to deep fascia
   (B) this is epicarnius muscle
   (C) muscle of facial expression
   (D) all of the above

4. Correct about occipitofrontalis is-
   (A) supplied by facial nerve
   (B) supplied by mandibular nerve
   (C) supplied by ophthalmic division of trigeminaaaal nerve
   (D) all of the above

5. Surgical scalp is made up of-
   (A) skin & connective tissue
   (B) skin, connective tissue & epicranial aponeurosis
   (C) skin, connective tissue, epicranial aponeurosis & loose areolar tissue
   (D) skin, connective tissue, epicra-nial aponeurosis & pericranium

6. Dangerous layer of scalp is-
   (A) connective tissue layer
   (B) loose areolar tissue layer
   (C) epicranial aponeurosis
   (D) pericranium

7. True about black eye is-
   (A) blood collects in loose areolar tissue layer
   (B) frontal belly has no bony attachment
   (C) common cause is head injury or direct injury to scalp
   (D) all of the above

8. Arteries supplying scalp in front of auricle are all except-
   (A) supratrochlear artery
   (B) supraorbital artery
   (C) superficial temporal artery
   (D) auriculo-temporal artery

9. All are branches of external carotid artery on scalp except-
(A) supratrochlear artery
(B) occipital artery
(C) superficial temporal artery
(D) posterior-auricular artery

10. Nerves supplying the scalp anterior to auricle are all except-
(A) supra trochlear n
(B) supraorbital n
(C) auriculotemporal n
(D) posterior auricular n

11. Nerves supplying the scalp posterior to auricle are all except-
(A) lesser occipital n
(B) greater occipital n
(C) auriculotemporal n
(D) great auricular n

12. Blood vessels and nerves supplying scalp anterior to auricle are -
(A) supratrochlear artery
(B) supra-orbital artery
(C) auriculotemporal nerves
(D) all of the above

13. Temporal lines are present on -
(A) temporal bone
(B) parietal bone
(C) sphenoid bone
(D) all of the above

14. Blood vessels and nerves supplying scalp posterior to auricle are all except-
(A) posterior auricular artery
(B) occipital artery
(C) great auricular nerves
(D) all of the above

15. Motor supply of scalp is-
(A) temporal branch facial nerve
(B) posterior auricular branch of facial n
(C) auriculo-temporal nerve
(D) A+B

16. Lymphatic drainage of scalp is-
(A) pre auricular lymph nodes
(B) posterior auricular lymph nodes
(C) occipital lymph nodes
(D) all of the above

17. Superficial surface of temporal fascia is related to all except-
(A) superficial temporal vessels
(B) deep temporal nerves
(C) Auriculotemporal nerve
(D) temporal branch of facial nerve

18. True about temporal fascia is –
(A) thickest fascia of the body
(B) morphologically represents bone
(C) used for tympanoplasty
(D) all of the above

19. True about face is-
(A) deep fascia contains muscle of facial expression
(B) muscles are derived from second branchial arch
(C) muscles of facial expression take origin from skin of the face
(D) all are true

20. Characteristic features of muscles of facial expression are –
(A) develop from 2nd branchial arch
(B) supplied by 7th cranial nerve
(C) lie in superficial fascia
(D) all of the above

21. Modiolus of angle of mouth is made up by-
(A) levatoranguli oris, zygomaticus major,
(B) levatoranguli oris, zygomaticus major & buccinator
(C) levatoranguli oris, zygomaticus major, risorius & buccinator
(D) levatoranguli oris, zygomaticus major, buccinator, depressor anguli oris & risorius

22. Muscles for- anger is-
(A) dilator naris
(B) dilator naris & depressor septi
(C) dilator naris, depressor septi & depressor anguli oris
(D) none of the above

23. Muscles responsible for frowning –
(A) corrugator supercilli + frontalis
(B) procerus + corrugator supercilli
(C) frontalis + procerus
(D) all of the above

24. Surprise or horror is expressed by-
(A) corrugator supercilli
(B) frontalis
(C) procerus
(D) none of the above

25. Muscle responsible for laughing-
(A) zygomaticus minor
(B) zygomaticus major
(C) risorius
(D) all of the above

26. Muscle responsible for disdain/doubt-
(A) risorius
(B) mentalis
(C) depressor labii inferioris
(D) none of the above

27. Worry is expressed by-
(A) depressor labii inferioris
(B) orbicularis occuli
(C) depressor septi
(D) all of the above

28. Cervical branch of facial nerve supplies-
(A) depressor labii inferioris
(B) platysma
(C) depressor septi
(D) all of the above

29. Zygomatic branch of facial nerve supplies-
(A) upper part of orbicularis oculi
(B) lower part of orbicularis oculi
(C) frontalis
(D) corrugator supercilli

30. Temporal branch of facial nerve supplies-
(A) upper part of orbicularis oculi
(B) frontalis
(C) corrugator supercilli
(D) all of the above

31. Marginal mandibular branch of facial nerve supplies-
(A) risorius
(B) depressor anguli oris + deprosser labii inferioris
(C) mentalis
(D) all of the above

32. Lower buccal branch of facial nerve supplies-
(A) risorius + orbicularis oris
(B) depressor anguli oris + buccinator
(C) orbicularis oris + buccinator + muscles of nose
(D) orbicularis oris + buccinator

33. Upper buccal branch of facial nerve supplies-
(A) zygomaticus major & minor
(B) buccinator
(C) orbicularis oris + buccinator + muscles of nose
(D) all of the above

34. Mentalis muscle is supplied by-
(A) mental nerve
(B) marginal mandibular nerve
(C) cervical branch of facial nerve
(D) great auricular nerve

35. In bell's palsy –
(A) upper half of face is paralysed
(B) ipsilateral complete half of face is paralysed
(C) ipslateral upper half of face is paralysed
(D) ipsilateral lower half of face is paralysed

36. In supra nuclear facial nerve palsy –
(A) upper half of face is paralysed
(B) contrlateral lower half of face is paralysed
(C) contrlateral upper half of face is paralysed
(D) ipsilateral lower half of face is paralysed

37. In nuclear facial nerve palsy –
(A) upper half of face is paralysed
(B) upper half of face is not paralysed
(C) contrlateral upper half of face is paralysed
(D) ipsilateral lower half of face is paralysed

38. True about nerve supply of face-
(A) facial nerve is motor
(B) trigeminal nerve is sensory
(C) angle of jaw is supplied by C2&C3
(D) all of the above

39. All are branches from ophthalmic division of trigeminal nerve on face except
(A) supraorbital n
(B) supratrochlear n
(C) infraorbital n
(D) lacrimal n

40. All are branches from ophthalmic division of trigeminal nerve on face except
(A) lacrimal n
(B) infra trochlear n
(C) zygomaticofacial n
(D) external nasal n

41. All are branches from maxillary division of trigeminal nerve on face except-
(A) infraorbital n
(B) auriculotemporal n
(C) zygamaticofacial n
(D) zygamoticotemporal n

42. All are branches from mandibular divi sion of trigeminal nerve on face except
(A) buccal n
(B) marginal mandibular n
(C) auriculotemporal n
(D) mental n

43. Infra-orbital nerve is a branch of-
(A) opthalmic nerve
(B) maxillary nerve
(C) mandibular nerve
(D) facial nerve

44. Auriculotemporal nerve is a branch of-
(A) opthalmic nerve
(B) maxillary nerve
(C) mandibular nerve
(D) facial nerve

45. External nasal nerve is a branch of-
(A) opthalmic nerve
(B) maxillary nerve
(C) mandibular nerve
(D) facial nerve

46. Marginal mandibular nerve is a branch of-
(A) opthalmic nerve
(B) maxillary nerve
(C) mandibular nerve
(D) facial nerve

47. Buccinator is supplied by-
(A) opthalmic nerve
(B) maxillary nerve
(C) mandibular nerve
(D) facial nerve

48. Mucosa & skin over buccinator muscle is supplied by-
(A) opthalmic nerve
(B) maxillary nerve
(C) mandibular nerve
(D) facial nerve

49. All are true about facial artery except-
(A) arises in the neck at the level of greater cornu of hyoid bone
(B) branch of external carotid artery
(C) enters face at anterioinferior angle of masseter
(D) all of the above

50. Trigeminal neuralgia-
(A) sudden attack of pain in the distribution of trigeminal nerve
(B) mostly affects maxillary division
(C) also called tic dolourex
(D) all are true

51. Transverse facial artery-
(A) branch of superficial temporal artery
(B) emerges through parotid gland
(C) accompanied by buccal nerve
(D) all are true

52. Facial vein-
(A) formed by union of supraorbital & supratrochlear veins
(B) joins anterior division of retromandibular vein to form common facial vein
(C) common facial vein drains into internal jugular vein
(D) all are correct

53. Retro mandibular vein –
(A) Formed by union of maxillary & superficial temporal veins
(B) formed in the parotid gland
(C) posterior division joins posterior auricular vein to form external jugular vein
(D) all of the above

54. Dangerous area of face-
(A) upper lip & lower ½ of nose
(B) lower lip & upper ½ of nose
(C) upper & lower lip
(D) upper lip & nose

55. Lymphatics from lateral forehead & lateral half of eye lids drain into-
(A) pre auricular lymph nodes
(B) submandibular lymph nodes
(C) submental lymph nodes
(D) deep cervical group of lymph nodes

56. Lymphatics from central forehead, medial half of eye lids & nose drain into-
(A) pre auricular lymph nodes
(B) submandibular lymph nodes
(C) submental lymph nodes
(D) deep cervical group of lymph nodes

57. Lymphatics from central part of the lower lip & chin drain into-
(A) pre auricular lymph nodes
(B) submandibular lymph nodes
(C) submental lymph nodes
(D) deep cervical group of lymph nodes

58. Eye lashes are seen in-
(A) medial 5/6th
(B) lateral 5/6th
(C) medial 1/6th
(D) lateral 1/6th

59. Nasolacrimal duct is-
(A) endodermal in origin
(B) mesodermal in origin
(C) ectodermal in origin
(D) none of the above

60. Meibomian glands are-
(A) modified sebaceous glands
(B) located on the deep surface of tarsal plate
(C) arranged in single row-ducts open behind eyelashes in a single row
(D) all of the above

61. Tarsal glands -
(A) secret oily fluid to decrease evaporation of tears
(B) are sebaceous glands
(C) called as Meibomian glands
(D) all are true

62. True about glands of eyelids is-
(A) gland of zies-sebaceous gland
(B) gland of moll-sweat gland
(C) meibomian gland-sebaceous gland
(D) all of the above

63. Lymphatics from eyelids –
(A) medial ½ drain into-submandibular lymph nodes
(B) lateral ½ drains into–preauricular lymph nodes
(C) submental lymph nodes
(D) A & B

64. Glands of Moll are-
(A) modified sebaceous glands
(B) modified sweat glands
(C) modified salivary glands
(D) all of the above

65. Modified sebaceous glands in eyelids –
(A) gland of moll & zies
(B) gland of moll & meibomian
(C) gland of meibomian & zies
(D) all of the above

66. Nictitating membrane is represented in human eye-
(A) lacus lacrimalis
(B) plica semilunaris
(C) whitnail's tubercle
(D) all of the above

67. True about blood supply of eyelids is-
(A) from palpebral conjunctiva -facial vein
(B) from bulbar conjunctiva-ophthalmic veins
(C) conjunctiva is supplied by ophthalmic artery
(D) all of the above

68. Superior palpebral conjunctiva is supplied by-
(A) optic nerve
(B) olfactory nerve
(C) opthalmic nerve
(D) maxillary nerve

69. Inferior palpebral conjunctiva is supplied by-
(A) optic nerve
(B) olfactory nerve
(C) opthalmic nerve
(D) maxillary nerve

70. True about the nerve supply of conjunctiva is-
(A) superior palpebral conjunctiva-opthalmic nerve
(B) ocular conjunctiva-opthalmic nerve
(C) inferior palpebral conjunctiva-maxillary nerve
(D) all of the above

71. Lacrimal gland is-
(A) J shaped serous gland
(B) large orbital & small palpebral part
(C) about a dozen of ducts
(D) all of the above

72. Orbital & palpebral part of lacrimal gland are separated by-
(A) tarsal plate
(B) levator palpebrae superioris
(C) orbicularis occuli
(D) all of the above

73. True about accessory lacrimal glands-
(A) called gland of Krause
(B) small serous glands beneath palpebral conjunctiva
(C) about 36 in upper & 6-8 in lower lid
(D) all of the above

74. Secretmotor fibers for lacrimation-
(A) lacrimatory nucleus is in medulla
(B) pass through nervus intermedius
(C) both a + b
(D) none of the above

75. True about preganglionic secretomotor supply for lacrimal gland-
(A) lacrimatory nucleus in pons
(B) nervus intermedius-geniculate ganglion- greater petrosal nerve
(C) nerve of pterygoid canal-pterygopaltine ganglion
(D) all are true

76. True about postganglionic secreto-motor supply for lacrimal gland-
(A) pterygopalatine ganglion
(B) maxillary nerve-zygomatic branch-zygomaticotemporal nerve
(C) lacrimal nerve-lacrimal gland
(D) all are true

77. Dangerous area of scalp is-
(A) connective tissue layer
(B) epicranial aponeurosis
(C) loose areolar tissue
(D) pericranium

78. Lower lip gets sensory supply by-
(A) buccal branch of facial nerve
(B) marginal mandibular branch of facial nerve
(C) mental nerve
(D) buccal branch of mandibular nerve

79. Buccinator muscle is supplied by-
(A) masseteric branches of mandibular nerve
(B) marginal mandibular branch of facial nerve
(C) buccal branch of facial nerve
(D) buccal branch of mandibular nerve

Answersheet

1. C, 2. A, 3. D, 4. A, 5. B, 6. B, 7. D, 8. D, 9. A, 10. D, 11. C, 12. D, 13. B, 14. D, 15. D, 16. D, 17. B, 18. D, 19. B, 20. D, 21. D, 22. B, 23. B, 24. B, 25. B, 26. B, 27. B, 28. B, 29. B, 30. D, 31. D, 32. D, 33. A, 34. B, 35. B, 36. B, 37. D, 38. D, 39. C, 40. C, 41. B, 42. B, 43. B, 44. C, 45. A, 46. D, 47. D, 48. C, 49. D, 50. D, 51. D, 52. D, 53. D, 54. A, 55. A, 56. B, 57. C, 58. B , 59. C, 60. D, 61. D, 62. D, 63. D, 64. B, 65. C, 66. B, 67. D, 68. C, 69. D, 70. D, 71. D, 72. B, 73. D, 74. B, 75. D, 76. D, 77. C, 78. C, 79. C

Chapter 3

Cranial Cavity

1. In adults bones of skull cap are having-
   (A) outer table of compact bone
   (B) inner table of compact bone
   (C) middle layer of spongy bone called diploe
   (D) all of the above

2. In children bones of cranial vault are-
   (A) triple layered
   (B) double layered
   (C) single layered
   (D) none of the above

3. Floor of anterior cranial fossa is formed by all except-
   (A) frontal
   (B) ethmoid
   (C) dorsum sella
   (D) sphenoid

4. Structures passing through anterior ethmoidal foramen are all except-
   (A) anterior ethmoidal nerve- branch of nasociliary nerve
   (B) anterior ethmoidal artery-branch of ophthalmic artery
   (C) anterior ethmoidal nerve- branch oh nasopalatine nerve
   (D) anterior ethmoidal vein- tributary of ophthalmic vein

5. Structures passing through posterior ethmoidal foramen are all except-
   (A) posterior ethmoidal nerve- branch of nasociliary nerve
   (B) posterior ethmoidal artery-branch of ophthalmic artery
   (C) posterior ethmoidal nerve- branch oh nasopalatine nerve
   (D) posterior ethmoidal vein- tributary of ophthalmic vein

6. Middle cranial fossa is formed by-
   (A) body of sphenoid
   (B) greater wings of sphenoid
   (C) temporal bone petrous & squamous part
   (D) all of the above

7. Carotico-clenoid foramen or canal may be formed by-
   (A) anterior clenoid process & optic canal
   (B) anterior clenoid process & middle clenoid process
   (C) middle clenoid process & posterior clenoid process
   (D) anterior clenoid process & posterior clenoid process

8. Superior orbital fissure is bounded by-
(A) body & lesser wing of sphenoid
(B) body & greater wing of sphenoid
(C) greater & lesser wing of sphenoid
(D) body, lesser wing & greater wing of sphenoid

9. Foramen rotundum leads into-
(A) infratemporal fossa
(B) pterygo palatine fossa
(C) infra orbital foramen
(D) temporal fossa

10. Structures passing through optic canal-
(A) optic nerve, ophthalmic artery
(B) optic nerve, ophthalmic artery & sympathetic plexus
(C) optic nerve, piamater, arachnoid mater, ophthalmic artery & sympathetic plexus
(D) optic nerve, pia, arachnoid; duramater ophthalmic artery & sympathetic plexus

11. Structures passing through superior orbital fissure – via ring of zinn
(A) occulomotor nerve & nasociliary nerve
(B) trochlear nerve & nasociliary nerve
(C) occulomotor n, abduscent n & nasociliary n
(D) occulomotor n, abduscent n & trochlear n

12. Structures passing through upper lateral part of superior orbital fissure –
(A) occulomotor nerve & nasociliary nerve
(B) trochlear nerve, frontal & nasociliary nerve
(C) trochlear, frontal & lacrimal nerve
(D) occulomotor n, abduscent n & trochlear n

13. Structures passing through inferior part of superior orbital fissure –
(A) superior ophthalmic vein & lacrimal artery
(B) trochlear nerve & inferior ophthalmic vein
(C) inferior ophthalmic vein
(D) occulomotor n & superior ophthalmic vein

14. Structures passing through foramen ovale are all except-
(A) mandibular nerve
(B) accessory middle meningeal artery
(C) middle meningeal artery
(D) lessor petrosal nerve

15. Posterior cranial fossa is formed by-
(A) sphenoid, temporal & occipital
(B) sphenoid, temporal & parietal
(C) sphenoid, temporal, parietal & occipital
(D) none of the above

16. Structures passing through jugular foramen-
(A) anterior part-inferior petrosal sinus
(B) posterior part-sigmoid sinus
(C) middle part-9th, 10th & 11th cranial nerves
(D) all are true.

17. Structures passing through anterior condylar canal-
(A) hypoglossal nerve
(B) 12th cranial nerve & meningeal br of ascending pharyngeal artery
(C) 11th & 12th cranial nerves
(D) all of the above

18. Anterior part of foramen magnum gives way to-
(A) apical ligament of dens
(B) upper part of cruciform ligament
(C) membrane tectoria
(D) all of the above

19. Posterior part of foramen magnum gives way to all except-
(A) medulla oblongata with spinal root of accessory nerves
(B) 1 anterior & 2 posterior spinal arteries
(C) 2 vertebral arteries
(D) basilar artery

20. Venous sinuses enclosed in falx cerebri are all except-
(A) superior sagittal sinus
(B) inferior sagittal sinus
(C) occipital sinus
(D) straight sinus

21. Venous sinuses enclosed in tentorium cerebelli are all except-
(A) transverse sinus
(B) inferior petrosal sinus
(C) occipital sinus
(D) straight sinus

22. Venous sinuses enclosed in falx cerebelli is/are -
(A) transverse sinus
(B) inferior petrosal sinus
(C) occipital sinus
(D) straight sinus

23. Supratentorial dura is supplied by-
(A) ophthalmic nerve
(B) maxillary nerve
(C) nerves spinosus
(D) all of the above

24. Durameter in anterior cranial fossa is supplied by all except-
(A) ophthalmic nerve
(B) anterior ethmoidal nerve
(C) posterior ethmoidal nerve
(D) maxillary nerve

25. Durameter in middle cranial fossa is supplied by -
(A) ophthalmic nerve
(B) maxillary nerve
(C) recurrent branch of mandibular nerve
(D) B+C both

26. Durameter of posterior cranial fossa is supplied by -
(A) meningeal branches of vagus nerve
(B) meningeal branches of hypoglossal nerve (C1 & C2)
(C) cervical plexus
(D) all of the above

27. All are paired cranial sinuses except-
(A) cavernous venous sinus
(B) superior petrosal sinus
(C) anterior intercavernous sinus
(D) sphenoparietal sinus

28. False statement about cavernous venous sinus is-
(A) roof is formed by meningeal layer of dura
(B) floor is formed by meningeal layer of dura
(C) lateral wall is formed by meningeal layer of dura
(D) medial wall is formed by meningeal layer of dura

29. All relations of cavernous sinus are true except-
(A) superior-optic tract
(B) lateral-trigeminal ganglion
(C) anterior –supraorbital foramen
(D) posterior-apex of petrous temporal bone

30. Structures passing through lateral wall of cavernous sinus are all except-
(A) abduscent nerve
(B) trochlear nerve
(C) ophthalmic nerve
(D) maxillary nerve

31. Nerve passing through central part of cavernous sinus is-
(A) abduscent nerve
(B) trochlear nerve
(C) ophthalmic nerve
(D) maxillary nerve

32. Tributaries of cavernous sinus from orbit are –
(A) superior ophthalmic vein
(B) inferior ophthalmic vein
(C) central vein of retina
(D) all of the above

33. Tributaries of cavernous sinus from meninges is/are –
(A) sphenoparietal sinus
(B) middle meningeal vein
(C) both of above
(D) none of the above

34. All are communications of cavernous venous sinus except-
(A) internal jugular vein
(B) transverse sinus
(C) pterygoid sinus
(D) sphenoparietal sinus

35. Tributaries of superior sagittal sinus are-
(A) superior cerebral vein
(B) inferior ophthalmic vein
(C) veins of frontal air sinus
(D) parietal emissary veins

36. Tributaries of sigmoid sinus are-
(A) mastoid and condylar veins
(B) cerebellar veins
(C) internal auditory veins
(D) all of the above

37. Deepest cranial fossa is-
(A) Anterior cranial fossa
(B) middle cranial fossa
(C) posterior cranial fossa
(D) all of the above

38. Most commonly fractured cranial fossa is-
(A) anterior cranial fossa
(B) middle cranial fossa
(C) posterior cranial fossa
(D) none of the above

39. Largest diploic vein is-
(A) frontal diploic vein
(B) parietal diploic vein
(C) occipital diploic vein
(D) none of the above

40. True about cranial venous sinuses is –
(A) 7 paired sinuses
(B) 7 unpaired sinuses
(C) total 21 venous sinuses
(D) all are true

Answersheet

1. D, 2. C, 3. C, 4. C, 5. C, 6. D, 7. B, 8. D, 9. B, 10. D, 11. C, 12. C, 13. C, 14. C, 15. C, 16. D, 17. B, 18. D, 19. D, 20. C, 21. C, 22. C, 23. D, 24. A, 25. D, 26. D, 27. C, 28. B, 29. C, 30. A, 31. A, 32. D, 33. C, 34. D, 35. B, 36. D, 37. C, 38. B, 39.C, 40. D

Chapter 4

Root of Neck

1. Smallest of sclaneus muscle is-
(A) sclaneus anterior
(B) sclaneus medius
(C) sclaneus posterior
(D) none of the above

2. Longest and largest of sclaneus muscle is-
(A) sclaneus anterior
(B) sclaneus medius
(C) sclaneus posterior
(D) none of the above

3. Most superficial of sclaneus muscle is-
(A) sclaneus anterior
(B) sclaneus medius
(C) sclaneus posterior
(D) none of the above

4. Largest cervical sympathetic ganglia is-
(A) superior cervical ganglion
(B) middlle cervical ganglion
(C) inferior cervical ganglion
(D) all are of same size

5. All are true about cervical ganglion except-
(A) superior cervical ganglion lies in front of transverse process of C2 & C3
(B) middle cervical ganglion lies in front of transverse process of C4 & C5
(C) middle cervical ganglion lies in front of transverse process of C6
(D) inferior cervical ganglion lies in front of transverse process of C7

6. All are boundaries of sclaneo-vertebral triangle -
(A) medial-longus colli
(B) lateral-sclaneus anterior
(C) base- subclavian artery 1st part
(D) all of the above

7. Contents of sclaneo-vertebral triangle are-
(A) first part of vertebral artery
(B) thyrocervical trunk & inferior thyroid artery
(C) stellate ganglion
(D) all of the above

8. Boundaries of scalene triangle-
(A) base-first rib
(B) sclanes anterior –anteriorly & sclaneus medius -posteriorly
(C) subclavian artery passese through it
(D) all of the above

9. All are true about relations of sclaneus anterior muscle except-
(A) anterior- phrenic n, transverse & suprascapular artery
(B) anterior-anterior jugular & subclavian vein
(C) anterior-superior belly of omohyoid & sternocleidomastoid muscle
(D) anterior-carotid sheath with contents

10. All are true about relations of sclaneus anterior muscle except-
(A) posterior- subclavian artery & roots of brachial plexus
(B) posterior- cervical pleura
(C) posterior-subclavian vein
(D) posterior- sclaneus medius muscle

11. Root value of phrenic nerve is-
(A) C3 C4 C5
(B) C4 C5
(C) C4 C5 C6
(D) None of the above

12. Accessory phrenic nerve arises from-
(A) phrenic nerve
(B) branch from nerve to subclavius
(C) branch from supraclavicular nerves
(D) all of the above

13. Root value of accessory phrenic nerve is-
(A) C3
(B) C4
(C) C5
(D) C6

14. Distribution of phrenic nerve is-
(A) diaphragm
(B) diaphragmatic pleura
(C) pericardium
(D) all of the above

15. Longest prevertebral muscle is-
(A) rectus capitis anterior
(B) longus cervicis (colli)
(C) longus capitis
(D) rectus capitis lateralis

16. Second part of subclavian artery runs between sclaneus anterior and medius-
(A) along with upper trunk of brachial plexus
(B) along with middle trunk of brachial plexus
(C) along with lower trunk of brachial plexus
(D) none of the above

17. All are branches from 1st part of subclavian artery except-
(A) vertebral artery
(B) costocervical trunk
(C) thyrocervical trunk
(D) internal thoracic artery

18. Largest branch of 1st part of subclavian artery is-
(A) inferior thyroid artery
(B) vertebral artery
(C) thyrocervical trunk
(D) internal thoracic artery

19. All are branches from thyrocervical trunk except-
(A) inferior thyroid artery
(B) suprascapular artery
(C) transverse scapular artery
(D) deep cervical artery

20. Vertebral artery passes through foramen transversarium of-
(A) C7 – C1
(B) C6 -- C1
(C) C7 – C2
(D) T1 – C1

21. Shortest branch of subclavian artery is-
(A) inferior thyroid artery
(B) vertebral artery
(C) thyrocervical trunk
(D) internal thoracic artery

22. Costocervical trunk arises from-
(A) 1st part of subclavian artery on left side
(B) 2nd part of subclavian artery on right side
(C) A & B are correct
(D) none of the above

23. Dorsal scapular artery is a branch from subclavian artery-
(A) 1st part
(B) 2nd part
(C) 3rd part
(D) none of the above

24. All are anterior branches of external carotid artery except-
(A) superior thyroid artery
(B) lingual artery
(C) ascending pharyngeal artery
(D) facial artery

25. Most superficial part of subclavian artery is-
(A) 1st part
(B) 2nd part
(C) 3rd part
(D) 1st and 2nd part

26. Principal lymph node of Palatine tonsil is -
(A) jugulo-omohyoid lymph node
(B) jugulo-digastric lymph node
(C) supra clavicular lymph node
(D) paratracheal lymph node

27. Principal lymph node of Tongue is -
(A) jugulo-omohyoid lymph node
(B) jugulo-digastric lymph node
(C) supra clavicular lymph node
(D) paratracheal lymph node

28. Only unpaired lymph nodes in the neck cervical-collar is-
(A) parotid lymph nodes
(B) sub-mandibular lymph nodes
(C) sub-mental lymph nodes
(D) mastoid group of lymph nodes

29. Largest vein of neck is-
(A) external jugular vein
(B) internal jugular vein
(C) occipital vein
(D) anterior jugular vein

30. All drain into internal jugular vein except-
(A) inferior petrosal sinus
(B) lingual vein & facial vein
(C) superior thyroid vein
(D) posterior auricular vein

Answersheet

1. C, 2. B, 3. A, 4. A, 5. B, 6. D, 7. D, 8. D, 9. C, 10. C, 11. A, 12. B, 13. C, 14. D, 15. B, 16. C, 17. B, 18. B, 19. D, 20. B, 21. C, 22. C, 23. C, 24. C, 25. C, 26. B, 27. A, 28. C, 29. B, 30. D

Chapter 5

Triangles of Neck

1. All are true about anterior triangle of neck except -
   (A) base is formed by body of mandible
   (B) sternocleidomastoid forms posterior boundary
   (C) anterior boundary is formed by midline of neck
   (D) floor is formed by investing layer of deep cervical fascia

2. Sternocleidomastoid muscle is supplied by all except-
   (A) occipital artery
   (B) superior thyroid artery
   (C) inferior thyroid artery
   (D) suprascapular artery

3. Sternocleidomastoid muscle is crossed superficially by all except-
   (A) great auricular nerve
   (B) external jugular vein
   (C) internal jugular vein
   (D) transrverse cervical nerve

4. Sternocleidomastoid muscle is related to all on deep surface except-
   (A) external carotid artery
   (B) 9th, 10th, 11th & 12th cranial nerves
   (C) external jugular vein
   (D) internal jugular vein

5. Roof of the posterior triangle is pierced by all except-
   (A) lesser occipital nerve
   (B) great auricular nerve
   (C) cranial accessory nerve
   (D) supraclavicular nerve

6. Roof of the posterior triangle is pierced by all except-
   (A) transerverse cervical nerve
   (B) external jugular vein
   (C) internal jugular vein
   (D) supraclavicular nerve

7. Floor of the posterior triangle is formed by -
   (A) semispinalis capitis
   (B) splenius capitis
   (C) levator scapulae
   (D) all of the above

8. All are contents of occipital triangle except-
   (A) external jugular vein
   (B) occipital artery
   (C) dorsal scapular nerve
   (D) spinal accessory nerve

9. All are contents of occipital triangle except-
(A) subclavian artery
(B) occipital artery
(C) supraclavicular nerves
(D) superficial transverse cervical artery

10. All are contents of supraclavicular triangle except-
(A) subclavian artery
(B) trunks of brachial plexus
(C) supraclavicular nerves
(D) superficial transverse cervical artery

11. All structures in posterior triangle of neck are deep to prevertebral fascia except-
(A) spinal accessory nerve
(B) occipital artery
(C) subclavian artery
(D) brachial plexus nerve

12. Boundaries of posterior triangle of neck are all except-
(A) posterior border of sternocleidomastoid
(B) anterior border of trapezius
(C) posterior 1/3 of clavicle
(D) middle 1/3 of clavicle

13. Boundaries of occipital triangle of neck are all except-
(A) posterior border of sternocleidomastoid
(B) anterior border of trapezius
(C) superior belly of omohyoid
(D) inferior belly of omohyoid

14. Boundaries of subclavian triangle of neck are all except-
(A) posterior border of sternocleidomastoid
(B) inferior belly of omohyoid
(C) anterior 1/3 of clavicle
(D) middle 1/3 of clavicle

15. Occasionally clavicle is pierced by –
(A) medial supraclavicular nerve
(B) middle supraclavicular nerve
(C) lateral supraclavicular nerve
(D) all of the above

16. During lymph node removal /biopsy in posterior triangle of neck nerve most commonly damaged is-
A lesser occipital nerve
(B) great auricular nerve
(C) spinal accessory nerve
(D) supraclavicular nerve

17. Virchow's lymph nodes are-
(A) right supraclavicular lymph nodes
(B) left supraclavicular lymph nodes
(C) right subclavicular lymph nodes
(D) left subclavicular lymph nodes

18. Commonest cause of cervical lymphadenopathy in children-
(A) cancer
(B) scalp infection
(C) cervical abscess
(D) meningitis

19. Commonest cause of cervical lymphadenopathy in adults-
(A) cancer
(B) scalp infection
(C) cervical abscess
(D) meningitis

20. Sternocleidomastoid is supplied by-
(A) spinal accessory nerve
(B) C2 & C3 nerve
(C) Both
(D) cranial accessory nerve

21. Spinal accessory nerve supplies –
(A) sternocleidomastoid + levator scapulae
(B) trapezius + levator scapulae
(C) sternocleidomastoid + trapezius
(D) levator scapulae + inferior belly of omohyoid

22. Sclaneus medius is pierced by-
(A) lesser occipital nerve
(B) great auricular nerve
(C) dorsal scapular nerve
(D) supraclavicular nerve

23. Trunks of brachial plexus pass between-
(A) sclaneus medius & sclaneus posterior
(B) sclaneus anterior & sclaneus posterior
(C) sclaneus anterior & sclaneus medius
(D) levator scapulae + inferior belly of omohyoid

24. Wrong srtatement is-
(A) subclavian vein passes posterior to sclaneus anterior
(B) subclavian artery passes posterior to sclaneus anterior
(C) lower trunk of brachial plexus passes posterior to sclaneus anterior
(D) subclavian vein passes anterior to sclaneus anterior

25. Transverse cervical artery –
(A) branch of thyrocervical trunk
(B) crosses sclaneus anterior & medius
(C) crosses upper trunk of brachial plexus
(D) all of the above

26. Most common cause of swelling in posterior triangle of neck-
(A) cystic hygroma
(B) potato tumor
(C) supraclavicular lymphadenopathy
(D) goiter

27. All are true about hyoid bone except-
(A) horse shoe shaped bone
(B) does not articulate with any bone
(C) lies at the level of C3
(D) develops from 1st branchial arch

28. Upper border of thyroid cartilage corresponds to-
(A) C2 vertebra
(B) C3 vertebra
(C) C4 vertebra
(D) C5 vertebra

29. Level of Cricoid cartilage corresponds to-
(A) C4 vertebra
(B) C5 vertebra
(C) C6 vertebra
(D) C7 vertebra

30. Investing layer of deep cervical fascia forms roof of-
(A) supraclavicular triangle
(B) carotid triangle
(C) both A&B
(D) none of the above

31. All are parts of anterior triangle except -
(A) digastric triangle
(B) carotid triangle
(C) subclavian triangle
(D) muscular triangle

32. All are complete triangles on one side of neck except-
(A) digastric triangle
(B) carotid triangle
(C) submental triangle
(D) muscular triangle

33. All are true for sub mental triangle except -
(A) body of hyoid forms base
(B) digastric muscles form sides
(C) base is formed by mandible
(D) floor is formed by mylohyoid

34. All are true for sub mental triangle except -
(A) body of hyoid forms base
(B) submental lymph nodes are content
(C) anterior belly of digastric muscles form side
(D) floor is formed by investing layer of deep cervical fascia

35. Submental lymph nodes drain all except-
(A) roof of mouth
(B) tip of the tongue
(C) floor of oral cavity
(D) lower incisor teeth

36. All are true for digastric triangle except -
(A) body of mandible forms base
(B) ant belly digastric form sides
(C) base is formed hyoid
(D) floor is formed by mylohyoid

37. Floor of digastric triangle is formed by all except -
(A) mylohyoid
(B) hyoglossus
(C) superior constrictor
(D) middle constrictor

38. Digastric triangle is divided by-
(A) stylohyoid ligament
(B) stylomandibular ligament
(C) styloglossus muscle
(D) stylohyoid muscle

39. Content of anterior part of digastric triangle are all except-
(A) carotid sheath with contents
(B) 12th cranial nerve
(C) submandibular gland
(D) facial artery

40. Content of anterior part of digastric triangle are all except-
(A) external carotid artery
(B) mylohyoid vessels & nerves
(C) facial artery & vein
(D) submental artery

41. Carotid triangle contains –
(A) external carotid artery
(B) internal carotid artery
(C) common carotid artery
(D) all of the above

42. Floor of carotid triangle is formed by all except -
(A) thyrohyoid
(B) hyoglossus
(C) superior constrictor
(D) middle constrictor

43. Carotid triangles contains all except-
(A) glossopharyngeal nerve
(B) vagus nerve
(C) accessory nerve
(D) hypoglossal nerve

44. Incorrect statement about carotid triangle is-
(A) post belly diagastric & stylohyoid forms antero superior boundary
(B) superior belly of omohyoid forms antero-inferior boundary
(C) floor is formed mylohyoid
(D) roof is formed by investing layer of deep cervical fascia

45. Common carotid artery bifurcates at the –
(A) upper border of cricoid
(B) upper border of thyroid
(C) lower border of thyroid
(D) none of the above

46. Artery not a content of carotid triangle is-
(A) ascending pharyngeal artery
(B) superior thyroid artery
(C) lingual artery
(D) posterior auricular artery

47. Artery not a content of carotid triangle is-
(A) facial artery
(B) inferior thyroid artery
(C) lingual artey
(D) occipital artery

48. 1st branch of external carotid artery is
(A) ascending pharyngeal artery
(B) superior thyroid artery
(C) lingual artery
(D) posterior auricular artery

49. All are anterior branches of external carotid artery except-
(A) facial artery
(B) maxillary artery
(C) lingual artey
(D) superior thyroid artery

50. Lingual artery arises at the level-
(A) tip of thyroid cartilage
(B) tip of greater cornu of hyoid bone
(C) tip of styloid process
(D) tip of lesser cornu of hyoid bone

51. Tributaries of internal jugular vein in carotid triangle are all except-
(A) facial vein
(B) common facial vein
(C) lingual vein
(D) superior thyroid vein

52. All are supra hyoid muscles except-
(A) stylohyoid
(B) mylohyoid
(C) geniohyoid
(D) omohyoid

53. Suprahyoid muscle is-
(A) digastric
(B) thyrohyoid
(C) sternothyroid
(D) omohyoid

54. Infrahyoid muscles are all except-
(A) stylohyoid
(B) thyrohyoid
(C) sternothyroid
(D) omohyoid

55. All are true for muscular triangle except-
(A) floor is formed by sternohyoid & sternothyroid
(B) contents are sternohyoid & sternothyroid
(C) floor is formed by deep cervical fascia
(D) roof is formed by deep cervical fascia

56. Laryngeal prominence –Adams apple is produced by-
(A) laryngeal cartilage
(B) thyroid cartilage
(C) cricoid cartilage
(D) none of the above

57. Thickest cutaneous nerve in head & neck -
(A) great auricular nerve
(B) greater occipital nerve
(C) lesser occipital nerve
(D) superficial temporal nerves

Answersheet

1. D, 2. C, 3. C, 4. C, 5. C, 6. C, 7. D, 8. A, 9. A, 10. C, 11. A, 12. C, 13. C, 14. C, 15. B, 16. C, 17. B, 18. B, 19. A, 20. C, 21. C, 22. C, 23. C, 24. A, 25. D, 26. C, 27. D, 28. C, 29. C, 30. C, 31. C, 32. C, 33. C, 34. D, 35. A, 36. C, 37. C, 38. B, 39. A, 40. A, 41. D, 42. C, 43. A, 44. C, 45. B, 46. D, 47. B, 48. A, 49. B, 50. B, 51. A, 52. D, 53. A, 54. A, 55. C, 56. B, 57. B

Chapter 6

Temporomandibular Joint

1. Grinning of face is produced by-
(A) mentalis
(B) risorius
(C) platysma
(D) zygomaticus major

2. Main lymph nodes of TMJ are
(A) submental lymph nodes
(B) submandibular lymph nodes
(C) parotid lymph nodes
(D) juglodigastric lymph nodes

3. TMJ is supplied by-
(A) Auriculotemporal n
(B) maxillary n
(C) greater auricular n
(D) all of the above

4. All are true for TMJ except-
(A) synovial, bicondylar variety
(B) articular surfaces are covered with fibrocartilages
(C) joint is displaced posteriorly commonly
(D) lateral pterygoid is inserted in the articular disc of joint

5. TMJ is supplied by-
(A) Auriculotemporal n
(B) massetric n
(C) both A & B
(D) Auriculotemporal n, massetric n & C1 from cervical plexus

6. Buccinators is supplied by-
(A) mandibular n
(B) facial n
(C) glossopharyngeal n
(D) nerve to mylohyoid

7. Retraction of mandible is done by-
(A) masseter
(B) lateral pterygoid
(C) temporalis
(D) medial pterygoid

8. Action of the lateral pterygoid muscle is-
(A) closing of mouth
(B) opening of mouth
(C) retraction of lower jaw
(D) clenching of the teeth

9. Most common cause of TMJ dislocation is-
(A) sudden closure of mouth
(B) blow on chin when mouth is closed
(C) blow on chin when mouth is widely open
(D) all of the above

10. All of the branches from posterior division of mandibular nerve are sensory except-
(A) mental nerve
(B) massetric nerve
(C) mylohyoid nerve
(D) none of the above

11. Most common nerve block in dental practice-
(A) lingual nerve
(B) inferior alveolar nerve
(C) mandibular nerve
(D) mylohyoid nerve

12. Most common direction of TMJ dislocation is-
(A) posterior
(B) anterior
(C) inferior
(D) postero-inferior

13. Muscle of head and neck called as Peripheral heart is-
(A) medial pterygoid
(B) lateral pterygoid
(C) medial & lateral pterygoid both
(D) temporalis

14. Chief elevator of jaw at TMJ is –
(A) temporalis
(B) masseter
(C) buccinators
(D) medial pterygoid

15. Largest division of trigeminal nerve is-
(A) mandibular division
(B) maxillary division
(C) ophthalmic division
(D) auriculo-temporal nerve

16. All are true about infra-temporal fossa except-
(A) located deep to ramus of mandible
(B) contains sub mandibular ganglion
(C) contains medial & lateral pterygoids
(D) communicates with pterygopalatine fossa

17. All are contents of infra-temporal fossa except-
(A) masseter muscle
(B) maxillary artery
(C) mandibular nerve
(D) chorda tympani nerve

18. All are true about roof of infratemporal fossa except-
(A) formed by greater wing of sphenoid
(B) pierced by foramen spinosum
(C) pierced by foramen rotendum
(D) pierced by foramen ovale

19. All pass through the roof of infratemporal fossa except-
(A) mandibular n
(B) middle meningeal artery
(C) maxillary nerve
(D) meningeal branch of mandibular n

20. All are true about infratemporal fossa except-
(A) roof-formed by greater wing of sphenoid
(B) medial wall- formed by ramus of mandible
(C) posterior wall – formed by styloid process
(D) lateral wall- formed by ramus of mandible

21. All are contents of infra temporal fossa except-
(A) lateral pterygoid
(B) masseter
(C) tendon of temporalis
(D) medial pterygoid

22. All are contents of infra temporal fossa except-
(A) mandibular nerve
(B) pterygoid venous plexus
(C) maxillary nerve
(D) maxillary artery

23. All are seen in infra temporal fossa except-
(A) otic ganglion
(B) chorda tympani nerve
(C) submandibular ganglion
(D) mandibular nerve

24. Infratemporal fossa communicates with all except-
(A) orbit
(B) oral cavity
(C) temporal fossa
(D) nasal cavity

25. All are true about communications of infratemporal fossa except-
(A) communicates with orbit through infra orbital fissure
(B) communicates with temporal fossa through deep to zygomatic arch
(C) communicates with nasal cavity through infra orbital fissure
(D) communicates with pterygopalatine fossa through pterygomaxillary fissure

26. All are true about lateral pterygoid except-
(A) it has two heads of origin
(B) supplied by posterior division of mandibular nerve
(C) inserted into neck of mandible & articular disc of TMJ
(D) opens the mouth or depresses the mandible

27. Superficial relations of Lateral pterygoid are all except-
(A) tendon of temporalis
(B) Maxillary nerve
(C) ramus of mandible
(D) superficial head of medial pterygoid

28. Deep relations of Lateral pterygoid are all except-
(A) mandibular n
(B) middle meningeal artery
(C) superficial head of medial pterygoid
(D) sphenomandibular ligament

29. All emerge through lower border of lateral pterygoid except-
(A) massetric nerves
(B) middle meningeal artery
(C) lingual nerve
(D) inferior alveolar nerve

30. Structures emerging through upper border of lateral pterygoid –
(A) massetric nerves
(B) deep temporal nerves
(C) Auriculotemporal nerve
(D) massetric & deep temporal nerves

31. Superficial relations of medial pterygoid are -
(A) lingual nerve
(B) inferior alveolar nerve
(C) inferior alveolar vessels
(D) all of the above

32. All are true about maxillary artery except-
(A) smaller terminal branch of External Carotid Artery
(B) arises behind neck of mandible
(C) related to lateral pterygoid
(D) enters the pterygo-palatine fossa through pterygo-maxillary fissure

33. All are branches of first part of maxillary artery except-
(A) deep auricular artery
(B) middle meningeal artery
(C) deep temporal arteries
(D) inferior alveolar artery

34. All are branches of second part of maxillary artery except-
(A) anterior tympanic artery
(B) deep temporal arteries
(C) massetric arteries
(D) pterygoid branches

35. All are branches of third part of maxillary artery except-
(A) posterior superior alveolar artery
(B) sphenopalatine artery
(C) deep auricular artery
(D) artery of pterygoid canal

36. True about muscles of mastication-
(A) develop from mesoderm of 1st branchial arch
(B) supplied by mandibular nerve
(C) all are inserted on the ramus of mandible
(D) all of the above

37. Acessory muscles of mastication are-
(A) digastric
(B) geniohyoid
(C) mylohyoid
(D) all of the above

38. Temporomandibular joint syndrome-
(A) diffuse facial pain –due to spasm of masseter muscle
(B) headache –due to spasm of temporalis muscle
(C) jaw ache-due to spasm of lateral pterygoids
(D) all of the above

39. Contents of pterygopalatine fossa are-
(A) maxillary nerve
(B) pterygopalatine ganglion
(C) maxillary artery 3rd part
(D) all of the above

40. True about pterygopalatine fossa is all except-
(A) contains maxillary nerve
(B) communicates with orbit through inferior orbital fissure
(C) ganglion of hay fever is a content
(D) maxillary 2nd part is a content

41. All are true for pterygopalatine fossa except-
(A) communicates with orbit anteriorly
(B) communicates with ptrygoid canal posteriorly
(C) communicates with nose medially
(D) communicates with infratemporal fossa inferіeriorly

42. Correct about pterygopalatine fossa is-
(A) communicates posteriorly with middle cranial fossa through foramen rotundum
(B) communicates posteriorly with pterygoid canal through foramen lacrerum
(C) communicates posteriorly with pharynx through palate-vaginal canal
(D) all of the above

43. All are correct about pterygo-palatine fossa except-
(A) communicates with oral cavity through graeter & lesser palatine canals
(B) communicates with nasal cavity through spheno-palatine foramen

(C) communicates with pharynx through palatovaginal canal

(D) communicates with middle cranial fossa through foramen lacerum

44. Maxillary nerve gives following branches in pterygo-palatine fossa except-

(A) ganglionic branches

(B) anterior superior alveolar nerve

(C) posterior superior alveolar nerve

(D) zygomatic nerve

45. Branches of maxillary nerve on face are all except-

(A) palpebral branch

(B) orbital branch

(C) nasal branch

(D) labial branch

46. All are true about inferior alveolar artery except-

(A) enters mandibular canal with inferior alveolar nerve

(B) branch of 1st part of maxillary artery

(C) branch of 3rd part of maxillary aretry

(D) inferior alveolar vein also accompanies artery

47. All are true about pterygoid venous plexus except-

(A) formed in and around medial pterygoid muscle

(B) formed in and around lateral pterygoid muscle

(C) drained into maxillary vein

(D) communicates to intracranial venous sinuses

48. Infratemporal fossa contains all except-

(A) mandibular nerve

(B) chorda tympani nerve

(C) otic ganglion

(D) trigeminal ganglion

49. All are true about auriculotemporal nerve except –

(A) arises from two roots and encircles middle meningeal artery

(B) supplies temporo-mandibular joint

(C) supplies submandibular salivary gland

(D) supplies external auditory meatus & tympanic membrane

50. Nerve to medial pterygoid supplies all except-

(A) medial pterygoid

(B) masseter

(C) tensor tympani

(D) tensor veli palati

51. Buccal branch of mandibular nerve supplies-

(A) buccinators muscle

(B) mucosa and skin covering buccinators muscle

(C) A + B

(D) none of the above

52. All are true about TMJ except-

(A) supplied by superficial temporal artery & maxillary artery

(B) supplied by superficial & deep temporal nerves

(C) supplied by auriculotemporal nerve

(D) supplied by massetric nerves

53. Most common nerve block given in dentistry is-

(A) lingual

(B) inferior alveolar

(C) mandibular

(D) all of the above

54. All of the muscles of mastication close the mouth except-
(A) temporalis
(B) masseter
(C) lateral pterygoid
(D) medial pterygoid

55. TMJ Dislocation are most common-
(A) posterior dislocation
(B) anterior dislocation
(C) medial dislocation
(D) postero-medial dislocation

56. Largest division of trigeminal nerve is-
(A) ophthalmic
(B) maxillary
(C) mandibular
(D) facial

57. Muscle of mastication so-called peripheral heart is-
(A) temporalis
(B) masseter
(C) lateral pterygoid
(D) medial pterygoid

58. Chief elevator of jaw is-
(A) temporalis
(B) masseter
(C) lateral pterygoid
(D) medial pterygoid

59. All are contents of pterygo-palatine fossa except-
(A) pterygo-palatine ganglion
(B) maxillary nerve
(C) 2nd part of maxillary artery
(D) 3rd part of maxillary artery

60. All are true about pterygo-palatine ganglion except-
(A) largest parasympathetic ganglion in head
(B) topographically related to maxillary nerve
(C) functionally related to facial nerve through lesser petrosal nerve
(D) secretomotor to lacrimal, nasal, palatal & pharyngeal glands

Answersheet

1. B, 2. C, 3. A, 4. C, 5. C, 6. B, 7. C, 8. B, 9. C, 10. C, 11. B, 12. B, 13. B, 14. B, 15. A, 16. B, 17. A, 18. C, 19. C, 20. B, 21. B, 22. C, 23. C, 24. B, 25. C, 26. B, 27. B, 28. C, 29. A, 30. D, 31. D, 32. A, 33. C, 34. A, 35. C, 36. D, 37. D, 38. D, 39. D, 40. D, 41. D, 42. D, 43. D, 44. B, 45. B, 46. C, 47. A, 48. D, 49. C, 50. B, 51. B, 52. B, 53. B, 54. C, 55. B, 56. C, 57. C, 58. B, 59. C, 60. C

Chapter 7

Salivary Glands

1. Largest salivary gland is
(A) sub mandibular gland
(B) parotid gland
(C) sublingual gland
(D) all of the above

2. Parotid gland is made up of –
(A) mucous acini mainly
(B) serous acini mainly
(C) serous + mucous acini
(D) all of the above

3. Parotid gland is related to all except-
(A) ramus of mandible anteriorly
(B) mastoid process posteriorly
(C) styloid process laterlly
(D) styloid process medially

4. Structure seprating parotid gland & submandibular gland is-
(A) parotid capsule
(B) styloglohyoid ligament
(C) stylomandibular ligament
(D) facial nerve

5. Structures entering or coming out from apex of parotid gland are-
(A) anterior division of retromandibular vein
(B) posterior division of retromandibular vein
(C) cervical branch of facial nerve
(D) all of the above

6. Structures entering or coming out from base of parotid gland are-
(A) superficial temporal artery
(B) Superficial temporal vein
(C) auriculo temporal nerve
(D) all of the above

7. Largest surface of parotid gland is-
(A) superficial or lateral surface
(B) anteromedial surface
(C) posteromedial surface
(D) base

8. Structures entering or comingout from posterior border of parotid gland are-
(A) posterior auricular artery
(B) posterior auricular vein
(C) posterior auricular branch of facial nerve
(D) all of the above

9. Contents of parotid gland are-
(A) facial nerve
(B) external carotid artery
(C) retromandibular vein
(D) all of the above

10. Most superficial structure in parotid gland is-
(A) retromandibular vein
(B) external carotid artery
(C) facial nerve
(D) all of the above

11. Most deep structure in parotid gland is-
(A) retromandibular vein
(B) external carotid artery
(C) facial nerve
(D) all of the above

12. Structure in the intermediate zone in parotid gland is-
(A) retromandibular vein
(B) external carotid artery
(C) facial nerve
(D) all of the above

13. Transverse facial artery is a branch of–
(A) superficial temporal artery
(B) maxillary artery
(C) external carotid artery
(D) facial artery

14. Parotid gland is divided into superficial & deep FACIOVENOUS plane by-
(A) retromandibular vein
(B) external carotid artery
(C) facial nerve
(D) all of the above

15. Parotid duct opens into vestibule of mouth-
(A) opposite to crown of 2nd mandibular premolar
(B) opposite to crown of 2nd mandibular molar
(C) opposite to crown of 2nd maxillary molar
(D) opposite to crown of 2nd maxillary premolar

16. Structures pierced by parotid duct are all except-
(A) buccal pad of fat & buccopharyngeal fascia
(B) buccinators muscle
(C) pharyngobasilar fascia
(D) buccal mucosa

17. Parotid gland is supplied by-
(A) auriculotemporal nerve + facial nerve
(B) great auricular nerve + facial nerve
(C) Auriculotemporal nerve+ great auricular nerve
(D) none

18. Parotid gland develops from-
(A) endoderm
(B) mesoderm
(C) ectoderm
(D) all

19. Cervicofacial trunks of facial nerve gives all branches except-
(A) temporal branch
(B) buccal branch
(C) cervical branch
(D) marginal mandibular branch

20. Secretomotor fibers to parotid gland are through-
(A) otic ganglion
(B) parotid ganglion
(C) submandibular ganglion
(D) pterygopalatine ganglion

21. Secretomotor nerve for parotid gland is –
(A) facial nerve
(B) glossopharyngeal nerve
(C) vagus nerve
(D) none of the above

22. Parotid gland start developing at-
(A) 6th week of intrauterine life
(B) 7th week of intrauterine life
(C) 8th week of intrauterine life
(D) 9th week of intrauterine life

23. Lymphatics draining parotid gland-
(A) superficial parotid lymph nodes
(B) deep parotid lymph nodes
(C) deep cervical lymph nodes
(D) all of the above

24. Commonest cause of parotid enlargement in children-
(A) measles
(B) mumps
(C) tumors
(D) sialolethiasis

25. Most common tumor of parotid gland-
(A) pleomorphic adenoma
(B) pott puffy tumor
(C) granuloma
(D) none of the above

26. Most preferred incision to drain parotid abscess-
(A) hilton's method
(B) sistrunk operation
(C) vertical incision
(D) none of the above

27. True about digastric muscle is all except-
(A) post belly is binnate
(B) ant belly is unipinnate
(C) both are inserted in intermediate tendon
(D) supplied by nerve to mylohyoid

28. Relations of posterior belly of diagastric are all except-
(A) carotid sheath with contents is deep
(B) posterior auricular artery & stylohyoid run on superior border
(C) occipital artery runs on lower border
(D) 10th, 11th & 12th cranial nerves are superficial

29. Action of mylohyoid muscle are all except-
(A) depress floor of mouth in deglutition
(B) elevates floor of mouth in deglutition
(C) depresses mandible against resistance
(D) elevates hyoid bone

30. Superficial relations of hyoglossus muscle are all except-
(A) lingual nerve
(B) glossopharyngeal nerve
(C) hypoglossal nerve
(D) deep part of submandibular gland

31. Superficial relations of hyoglossus muscle are all except-
(A) lingual nerve & submandibular ganglion
(B) lingual artery
(C) hypoglossal nerve
(D) styloglossus muscle

32. Deep relations of hyoglossus muscle are all except-
(A) genioglossus muscle
(B) lingual nerve
(C) glossopharyngeal nerve
(D) stylohyoid ligament

33. Structures passing deep to posterior border of hyoglossus muscle are all except-
(A) lingual artery
(B) lingual nerve
(C) glossopharyngeal nerve
(D) stylohyoid ligament

34. Lingual nerve arises from-
(A) trunk of mandibular nerve
(B) anterior division of mandibular nerve
(C) posterior division of mandibular nerve
(D) none of the above

35. Distribution of lingual nerve is-
(A) gingival branch for inner surface of gums
(B) secretomotor fibers to submandibular gland & sublingual gland
(C) branches to anterior 2/3 of the tongue
(D) all of the above

36. Hypoglossal nerve crosses all except while entering submandibular region-
(A) common carotid artery
(B) external carotid artery
(C) loop of lingual artery
(D) internal carotid artery

37. All are true about submandibular gland except-
(A) situated below and posterior to mylohyoid
(B) mixed type of salivary gland
(C) large superficial and a small deep part
(D) duct emerges from superficial part

38. Medial surface of superficial part of submandibular gland in anterior 1/3 is related to all except-
(A) mylohyoid
(B) hyoglossus
(C) mylohyoid nerves & vessels
(D) submental branch of facial artery

39. Medial surface of superficial part of submandibular gland in middle 1/3 is related to all except-
(A) hyoglossus
(B) mylohyoid
(C) lingual & hypoglossal nerves
(D) submandibular ganglion

40. Medial surface of superficial part of submandibular gland in posterior 1/3 is related to all except-
(A) stylohyoid ligament & styloglossus muscle
(B) hyoglossus
(C) glossopharyngeal nerves
(D) middle constrictor of pharynx

41. Lateral surface of superficial part of submandibular gland is related to all except-
(A) submandibular fossa on inner aspect of body of mandible
(B) mylohyoid
(C) facial artery
(D) medial pterygoid muscle

42. True about deep part of submandibular gland is all except-
(A) medially- hyoglossus muscle
(B) superior- lingual nevre & submandibular ganglion
(C) inferior- glossopharyngeal nerve
(D) laterally- mylohyoid muscle

43. All are true about submandibular duct except-
(A) emerges from anterior end of superficial part
(B) called as Wharton's duct
(C) runs on hyoglossus muscle between lingual nerve & hypoglossal nerve
(D) opens in mouth below tongue on sublingual papilla at the side of lingual frenulum

44. Lymphatic drainage of submandibular gland is-
(A) juglo-digastric lymph nodes
(B) juglo-omohyoid lymph nodes
(C) submental lymph nodes
(D) preauricular lymph nodes

45. Secretomotor nerve supply to submandibular gland comes through-
(A) submandibular ganglion
(B) langley's ganglion
(C) meckel's ganglion
(D) pterygopalatine ganglion

46. Secretomotor nerve supply to submandibular gland comes through lingual anatomically but functionally it is by -
(A) mandibular nerve
(B) facial nerve
(C) glossopharyngeal nerve
(D) maxillary nerve

47. All are true about sublingual gland except-
(A) smallest salivary gland,
(B) lies under the oral mucosa above oral diaphragm in sublingual fossa
(C) mainly serous in nature
(D) sub-mandibular ganglion is secretomotor for sublingual gland

48. Superficial relations of hyoglossus muscle are all except-
(A) lingual nerve
(B) glossopharyngeal nerve
(C) hypoglossal nerve
(D) deep part of submandibular gland

49. True about of salivary gland is-
(A) parotid- pyramidal shaped- 15 gms - ectodermal
(B) submandibular-J shaped- 7.5 gms – endodermal
(C) sublingual -almond shaped- 3-4 gms - endodermal
(D) all are true

50. Duct of Rivinus is-duct of-
(A) lacrimal gland
(B) submandibular gland
(C) sublingual gland
(D) accessory salivary glands

51. Nerve most commonly damaged in submandibular gland surgeries is-
(A) hypoglossal nerve
(B) glossopharyngeal nerve
(C) lingual nerve
(D) any of the above

52. Artery most commonly damaged in submandibular gland surgeries is-
(A) external carotid artery
(B) lingual artery
(C) facial artery
(D) internal carotid artery

Answersheet

1. B, 2. B, 3. C, 4. C, 5. D, 6. D, 7. A, 8. D, 9. D, 10. C, 11. B, 12. A, 13. A, 14. C, 15. C, 16. C, 17. C, 18. C, 19. A, 20. A, 21. B, 22. A, 23. D, 24. B, 25. A, 26. A, 27. D, 28. D, 29. A, 30. B, 31. B, 32. B, 33. B, 34. C, 35. D, 36. A, 37. D, 38. B, 39. B, 40. B, 41. B, 42. C, 43. A, 44. A, 45. A, 46. B, 47. C, 48. B, 49. D, 50. C, 51. C, 52. C

Chapter 8

Thyroid Gland

1. Largest endocrine gland is-
(A) thyroid
(B) pituitary
(C) adrenal
(D) parathyroid

2. Functions of thyroid gland are regulation of –
(A) basal metabolic rate
(B) psychosomatic growth
(C) calcium metabolism
(D) all of the above

3. Thyroid gland is located in the neck opposite to-
(A) C3, C4, C5 vertebrae
(B) C4, C5, C6 vertebrae
(C) C5, C6, C7 vertebrae
(D) C5, C6, C7 & T1 vertebrae

4. Each lateral lobe of thyroid gland lies opposite to-
(A) 4 & 5 tracheal rings
(B) 5 & 6 tracheal rings
(C) 6 & 7 tracheal rings
(D) 5, 6 & 7 tracheal rings

5. Isthmus of thyroid gland lies opposite to-
(A) 3rd & 4th tracheal rings
(B) 2nd, 3rd & 4th tracheal rings
(C) 3rd, 4th & 5th tracheal rings
(D) 5th, 6th & 7th tracheal rings

6. Thyroid gland is larger in –
(A) adolescent children
(B) during menstruation
(C) during pregnancy
(D) all of the above

7. Levator glandulae thyroidae is attached to-
(A) cricoid
(B) hyoid
(C) both
(D) none

8. Suspensory ligament of berry is attached to-
(A) cricoid
(B) hyoid
(C) both
(D) none

9. All are true about capsules of thyroid gland except-
   (A) true capsule is formed by condensation of fibrous stroma of gland
   (B) false capsule is made up of pretracheal layer of deep fascia
   (C) venous plexus lies between true & false capsule
   (D) venous plexus lies beneath the true capsule

10. All are true about apex of thyroid gland except-
   (A) apex is directed upwards and laterally till oblique line of thyroid cartilage
   (B) it is limited by attachment of sternothyroid muscle
   (C) medially middle constrictor and laterally sternothyroid are in relation to apex
   (D) medially inferior constrictor and laterally sternothyroid are in relation to apex

11. Muscles attached to oblique line of thyroid cartilage are all except-
   (A) thyrohyoid
   (B) sternothyroid
   (C) middle constrictor
   (D) inferior constrictor

12. True about arterial supply of thyroid gland is all except-
   (A) superior thyroid artery is a branch of external carotid artery
   (B) inferior thyroid artery is a branch of subclavian artery
   (C) superior thyroid artery supplies upper 2/3rd of gland
   (D) inferior thyroid artery supplies lower 2/3rd of the gland

13. All are true about venous drainage of thyroid gland is except -
   (A) superior thyroid veins drain into IJV of respective side
   (B) middle thyroid veins drain into IJV of respective side
   (C) fourth thyroid veins or vein of Kocher Drains into IJV of respective side
   (D) inferior thyroid veins drain into brachiocephalic veins of respective side

14. Nerve supply of throid gland is-
   (A) vagus nerve
   (B) recurrent laryngeal nerve
   (C) superior, middle & inferior cervical sympathetic ganglion
   (D) all of the above

15. Lymphatics from thyroid drain into-
   (A) lower part of isthmus drains into retrosternal & brachiocephalic group of lymph nodes
   (B) upper part of gland drain into-prelaryngeal & juglodigastric lymph nodes
   (C) lower part drains into pretracheal & lymph nodes along recurrent laryngeal nerve
   (D) all of the above

16. Thyroid gland develops as endodermal thickening at-
   (A) during 2nd week of intrauterine life
   (B) during 3rd week of intrauterine life
   (C) during 4th week of intrauterine life
   (D) during 5th week of intrauterine life

17. Thyroid gland reaches its definitive position by-
   (A) during 5th week of intrauterine life
   (B) during 6th week of intrauterine life
   (C) during 7th week of intrauterine life
   (D) during 8th week of intrauterine life

18. Thyroid gland becomes functional by-

(A) during 2nd month

(B) during 3rd month

(C) during 4th month

(D) none of the above

19. Trachea extends –

(A) cricoid cartilage till sternal angle

(B) thyroid cartilage till sternal angle

(C) hyoid bone till sternal angle

(D) all of the above

20. Trachea extends –

(A) C6 vertebra till T4 vertebra

(B) C6 vertebra till T2 vertebra

(C) C6 till T6 vertebra

(D) all of the above

21. External diameter of trachea is-

(A) 1.5 cms in male & 1.2 cms in females

(B) 1.5 cms in both male & females

(C) 2 cms in males & 1.5 cms in females

(D) 2 cms in both males & females

22. Lumen of trachea in newborn is-

(A) 2 mm

(B) 3 mm

(C) 4 mm

(D) variable

23. Lumen of trachea remains almost same as of new born till –

(A) 1st year of age

(B) 2nd year of age

(C) 3rd year of age

(D) 4th year of age

24. Lumen of trachea after third year of life increases on a rate of-

(A) 2mm per year

(B) 3 mm per year

(C) 1 mm per year

(D) 4 mm per year

25. Lumen of trachea almost reaches its adult size by-

(A) 8-10 years of age

(B) 12-14 years of age

(C) 14 -16 years of age

(D) 16-18 years of age

26. True about cervical part of trachea is-

(A) supplied by inferior thyroid arteries

(B) veins drain into left brachiocephalic vein

(C) lymphatics drain into pre & para tracheal group

(D) all of the above

27. Most vascular endocrine gland in the body is-

(A) thyroid

(B) pancreas

(C) pituitary

(D) adrenal

28. Most common site of thyroglossal cyct is-

(A) suprahyoid

(B) subhyoid

(C) hyoid

(D) sublingual

29. Most common cause of hypoparathyroidism is-

(A) thyroidectomy

(B) drug reaction

(C) parathyroidectomy

(D) none of the above

30. Most preferred site of tracheostomy is-

(A) 2nd & 3rd tracheal rings

(B) 3rd & 4th tracheal rings

(C) 4th & 5th tracheal rings

(D) all of the above

Answersheet

1. A, 2. D, 3. D, 4. B, 5. B, 6. D, 7. B, 8. A, 9. C, 10. C, 11. C, 12. C, 13. D, 14. D, 15. D, 16. B, 17. C, 18. B, 19. A, 20. A, 21. C, 22. B, 23. C, 24. C, 25. B, 26. D, 27. A, 28. B, 29. A, 30. A

Chapter 9

Oral Cavity & Tongue

31. On protruding the tongue it deviates to one side, nerve involved is-
(A) trigeminal nerve
(B) facial nerve
(C) hypoglossal nerve
(D) lingual nerve

32. Anterior two-third of the tongue is formed by-
(A) cupola of his
(B) lingual swellings
(C) hypobranchial eminence
(D) all

33. Hypoglossal nerve is motor for all except-
(A) hyoglossus
(B) genioglossus
(C) palatoglossus
(D) all of the above

34. Tip of the tongue drains into-
(A) submental lymph nodes
(B) submandibular lymph nodes
(C) preauricular lymph nodes
(D) juglo omohyoid lymph nodes

35. Musculature of tongue is supplied by-
(A) lingual nerve
(B) inferior alveolar nerve
(C) hypoglossal nerve
(D) glossopharyngeal nerve

36. In Cancer of tongue pain radiates to ear because of-
(A) lingual nerve
(B) trigeminal nerve
(C) glossopharyngeal nerve
(D) hypoglossal nerve

37. Safety muscle of tongue is-
(A) hyoglossus
(B) genioglossus
(C) palatoglossus
(D) styloglossus

38. Posterior 1/3 of the tongue – sensory supply is-
(A) lingual nerve
(B) vagus nerve
(C) glossopharyngeal nerve
(D) hypoglossal nerve

39. Anterior 2/3 of the tongue –sensory supply is-
(A) lingual nerve
(B) vagus nerve
(C) glossopharyngeal nerve
(D) hypoglossal nerve

40. Anterior 2/3 of the tongue is supplied by-

(A) lingual nerve + chorda tympani nerve

(B) chorda tympani nerve + glossopharyngeal nerve

(C) glossopharyngeal nerve + vagus nerve

(D) none of the above

41. Anterior 2/3 of the tongue is supplied by-

(A) lingual nerve + chorda tympani nerve + hypoglossal nerve

(B) chorda tympani nerve + glossopharyngeal nerve + hypoglossal nerve

(C) glossopharyngeal nerve + vagus nerve + lingual nerve

(D) none of the above

42. Posterior 1/3 of the tongue is supplied by-

(A) lingual nerve + chorda tympani nerve

(B) chorda tympani nerve + glossopharyngeal nerve

(C) glossopharyngeal nerve + vagus nerve

(D) glossopharyngeal nerve + hypoglossal nerve

43. Posterior most part of tongue is supplied by-

(A) lingual nerve + chorda tympani nerve

(B) vagus nerve + glossopharyngeal nerve

(C) glossopharyngeal nerve + hypoglossal nerve

(D) vagus nerve+ hypoglossal nerve

44. Taste sensations from anterior 2/3 of the tongue is carried by-

(A) lingual nerve

(B) chorda tympani nerve

(C) glossopharyngeal nerve

(D) B+C

45. Taste sensations from posterior 1/3 of the tongue is carried by-

(A) lingual nerve

(B) chorda tympani nerve

(C) glossopharyngeal nerve

(D) hypoglossal nerve

46. Taste sensations from posterior most part of the tongue is carried by-

(A) lingual nerve

(B) chorda tympani nerve

(C) superior laryngeal nerve

(D) glossopharyngeal nerve

47. General & taste sensations from anterior 2/3 of tongue is carried by

(A) lingual nerve + chorda tympani nerve

(B) chorda tympani nerve + glossopharyngeal nerve

(C) lingual +chorda tympani nerve + glossopharyngeal nerve

(D) glossopharyngeal nerve + vagus + hypoglossal nerve

48. Circumvallate papilla present in anterior 2/3 rd of tongue are supplied by-

A lingual nerve

(B) chorda tympani

(C) glossopharyngeal nerve

(D) hypoglossal nerve

49. Retraction of the tongue is done by-

(A) genioglossus

(B) palatoglossus

(C) styloglossus

(D) hyoglossus

50. Protrusion of the tongue is done by-
(A) genioglossus
(B) palatoglossus
(C) styloglossus
(D) hyoglossus

51. Posterior part of the tongue is elevated by-
(A) genioglossus
(B) palatoglossus
(C) styloglossus
(D) hyoglossus

52. Depression of the tongue is done by-
(A) genioglossus
(B) palatoglossus
(C) styloglossus
(D) hyoglossus

53. All of the tongue muscles are supplied by-
(A) accessory spinal nerve
(B) nucleus ambiguss through pharyngeal plexus
(C) hypoglossal
(D) none of the above

54. Palatoglossus muscle of tongue is supplied by-
(A) hypoglossal
(B) accessory spinal
(C) accessory cranial
(D) all of the above

55. Tongue is supplied by –
(A) lingual arteries
(B) tonsillar branch of facial artery
(C) ascending pharyngeal artery
(D) all of the above

56. First tooth to erupt is-
(A) lower central incisior
(B) upper central incisior
(C) lateral incisior
(D) none of the above

57. First permanent tooth to appear is-
(A) medial incisior
(B) lateral incisior
(C) first molar
(D) first premolar

58. Tooth absent in children are-
(A) incisiors
(B) canine
(C) premolars
(D) molars

59. Bicuspid teeth are-
(A) molar
(B) premolar
(C) canine
(D) incisiors

60. Most common tooth to be unerupted and impacted is-
(A) 3rd premolar
(B) 3rd molar
(C) canine
(D) none of the above

61. safety muscle of the tongue is-
(A) genioglossus
(B) styloglossus
(C) palatoglossus
(D) hyoglossus

Answersheet

1. C, 2. B, 3. C, 4. A, 5. C, 6. C, 7. B, 8. C, 9. A, 10. A, 11. A, 12. D, 13. D, 14. D, 15. C, 16. C, 17. C, 18. C, 19. C, 20. A, 21. B, 22. D, 23. C, 24. C, 25. D, 26. A, 27. C, 28. C, 29. B, 30. B, 31. A

Chapter 10

Pharynx & Larynx

1. All are longitudinal muscles of pharynx except-
   (A) stylopharyngeus
   (B) thyropharyngeus
   (C) palatopharyngeus
   (D) salpingopharyngeus

2. Nasopharynx is supplied by-
   (A) pharyngeal branches from pterygopalatine ganglion-maxillary nerve
   (B) glossopharyngeal nerve
   (C) internal laryngeal nerve
   (D) all of the above

3. Oropharynx is supplied by-
   (A) pharyngeal branches from pterygopalatine ganglion-maxillary nerve
   (B) glossopharyngeal nerve
   (C) internal laryngeal nerve
   (D) all of the above

4. Laryngopharynx is supplied by-
   (A) pharyngeal branches from pterygopalatine ganglion-maxillary nerve
   (B) glossopharyngeal nerve
   (C) internal laryngeal nerve
   (D) all of the above

5. Pharynx is supplied by-
   (A) pharyngeal branches from pterygopalatine ganglion-maxillary nerve
   (B) glossopharyngeal nerve
   (C) internal laryngeal nerve
   (D) all of the above

6. Structures passing through sinus of Morgagni-
   (A) auditory tube
   (B) levator palate muscle
   (C) ascending palatine & palatine branch of ascending pharyngeal artery
   (D) all of the above

7. Sinus of Morgagni is space between-
   (A) between superior & middle constrictor
   (B) between inferior & middle constrictor
   (C) between skull & superior constrictor
   (D) betweencircular & longitudinal part of inferior constrictor

8. Structures passing through between superior & middle constrictor
(A) auditory tube
(B) levator palati muscle
(C) glossopharyngeal nerve & levator palate
(D) glossopharyngeal nerve & stylopharyngeus

9. Structures passing between middle & inferior constrictor-
(A) internal laryngeal nerve & inferior laryngeal artery
(B) superior laryngeal nerve & superior laryngeal artery
(C) external laryngeal nerve & superior laryngeal artery
(D) internal laryngeal nerve & superior laryngeal artery

10. Structures passing through inferior constrictor & oesophagus -
(A) recurrent laryngeal nerve & inferior laryngeal artery
(B) recurrent laryngeal nerve & superior laryngeal artery
(C) internal laryngeal nerve & superior laryngeal artery
(D) internal laryngeal nerve & inferior laryngeal artery

11. Pharyngeal plexus is located on-
(A) superior constrictor muscle
(B) middle constrictor muscle
(C) inferior constrictor muscle
(D) all of the above

12. Pharyngeal plexus of nerves is formed by-
(A) 9th & 10th cranial nerve
(B) 9th, 10th & 11th cranial nerve
(C) 9th, 10th & 11th cranial nerve & superior cervical sympathetic nerve
(D) 9th, 10th, 11th & 12th cranial nerve

13. Arterial supply of pharynx is from-
(A) lingual artery & facial artery
(B) lingual, facial & ascending pharyngeal artery
(C) lingual, facial, maxillary & ascending pharyngeal artery
(D) none of the above

14. Venous plexus of pharynx is located on-
(A) superior constrictor muscle
(B) middle constrictor muscle
(C) inferior constrictor muscle
(D) all of the above

15. Venous plexus of pharynx drains into-
(A) external jugular vein
(B) internal jugular vein
(C) maxillary vein
(D) none of the above

16. Palatine tonsils are situated in tonsillar fossa in –
(A) lateral wall of nasopharynx
(B) lateral wall of oropharynx
(C) lateral wall of laryngopharynx
(D) none of the above

17. All are true about tonsillar fossa except-
(A) anterior- palatoglossal arch
(B) posterior-palatopharyngeus
(C) apex-hard palate
(D) base- posterior third of tongue

18. All are true about tonsillar fossa except-
(A) anterior- palatoglossal arch
(B) posterior-palatopharyngeus
(C) tonsillar bed-middle constrictor
(D) apex- soft palate

19. Tonsillar bed is formed mainly by-
(A) superior constrictor muscle
(B) middle constrictor muscle
(C) inferior constrictor muscle
(D) all of the above

20. Tonsillar bed is formed mainly by-
(A) pharyngo basilar fascia
(B) superior constrictor muscle
(C) buccopharyngeal fascia
(D) all of the above

21. Structures seprated from tonsil by tonsillar bed are-
(A) facial artery
(B) styloglossus & glossopharyngeal nerve
(C) submandibular gland
(D) all of the above

22. Tonsil is fixed by suspensory ligament to-
(A) soft palate at upper pole
(B) posterior part of tongue to lower pole
(C) laterally with tonsillar bed
(D) all of the above

23. True about arterial supply of tonsil is-
(A) tonsillar branch of facial artery is main artery
(B) enters through lower pole
(C) pierces superior constrictor
(D) all of the above

24. Arterial supply of palatine tonsil is by-
(A) tonsillar & ascending palatine branch of facial artery
(B) dorsal lingual branch of lingual artery
(C) ascending pharyngeal branch of external carotid artery
(D) all of the above

25. Common source of bleeding after tonsillectomy is-
(A) tonsillar artery branch of facial artery
(B) paratonsillar vein
(C) pretonsillar vein
(D) none of the above

26. True about venous drainage of palatine tonsil is-
(A) drained into paratonsillar vein
(B) paratonsillar vein drains into pharyngeal plexus
(C) pharyngeal plexus of veins drains into internal jugular vein
(D) all of the above

27. Pharyngo-tympanic tube in adults is-
(A) 36 mm long
(B) directed downward, forwards & medially
(C) makes an angle of 45° with horizontal plane
(D) all are correct

28. True about pharyngo-tympanic tube in children is all except-
(A) 18 mm long
(B) directed downward, forwards & medially
(C) makes an angle of 10° with horizontal plane
(D) no angulation

29. True about eustachian tube is-
(A) lateral 1/3rd is bony
(B) medial 1/3rd is bony
(C) lateral 2/3rd is bony
(D) medial 2/3rd is bony

30. Cartilaginous part of auditory tube is-
(A) medial 2/3
(B) made up of single piece of elastic fibro cartilage
(C) 24 mm in length
(D) all of the above

31. Widest part of pharyngo tympanic tube is-
(A) tympanic end
(B) isthmus
(C) pharyngeal end
(D) none of the above

32. Most narrow part of pharyngo tympanic tube is-
(A) tympanic end
(B) pharyngeal end
(C) isthmus
(D) none of the above

33. Cartilage portion of pharyngo tympanic tube is-
(A) single piece of fibrocartilage
(B) forms medial wall & roof
(C) partly forms lateral wall
(D) all of the above

34. Incisive canal or foramen transmits-
(A) greater palatine nerve & greater palatine vessels
(B) naso-palatine nerve & greater palatine vessels
(C) lesser palatine nerve & greater palatine vessels
(D) greater palatine nerve & lesser palatine vessels

35. Greater palatine foramen transmits-
(A) greater palatine nerve & lesser palatine vessels
(B) greater palatine nerve & greater palatine vessels
(C) lesser palatine nerve & greater palatine vessels
(D) greater palatine nerve & lesser palatine vessels

36. Lesser palatine foramen transmits-
(A) greater palatine nerve & greater palatine vessels
(B) lesser palatine nerve & lesser palatine vessels
(C) lesser palatine nerve & greater palatine vessels
(D) greater palatine nerve & lesser palatine vessels

37. True about hard palate is-
(A) supplied by greater palatine artery
(B) veins drain into pterygoid plexus
(C) greater palatine & nasopalatine nerve
(D) all are ture

38. Intrinsic muscle of soft palate is-
(A) tensor veli palatini
(B) levator veli palatini
(C) musculus uvulae
(D) palatopharyngeus

39. Soft palate is supplied by all except-
(A) lesser palatine branch of maxillary artery
(B) ascending palatine branch of facial artery
(C) greater palatine branch of maxillary artery
(D) palatine branch of ascending pharyngeal artery

40. Tensor veli palatine is supplied by-
(A) pharyngeal plexus through vagus
(B) accessory cranial nerve through pharyngeal plexus
(C) mandibular nerve
(D) pterygopalatine ganglion

41. Largest tonsil is-
(A) tubal tonsil
(B) retropharyngeal tonsil
(C) palatine tonsil
(D) lingual tonsil

42. Larynx is situated in neck against-
(A) 3rd, 4th, 5th cervical vertebrae
(B) 3rd, 4th, 5th & 6th cervical vertebrae
(C) 4th, 5th & 6th cervical vertebrae
(D) 2nd, 3rd, 4th, 5th cervical vertebrae

43. In children & females larynx is located at -
(A) at lower level
(B) at higher level
(C) at the same level
(D) none of the above

44. All are unpaired cartilage of larynx except-
(A) thyroid
(B) arytenoid
(C) cricoid
(D) epiglottis

45. All are paired cartilage of larynx except-
(A) arytenoid
(B) cricoid
(C) corniculate
(D) cuneiform

46. Posterior surface of thyroid cartilage gives attachment to all except—
(A) thyroepiglottic ligament
(B) thyrohyoid ligament
(C) a pair of vestibular ligament
(D) a pair of vocal ligaments

47. Posterior border of thyroid cartilage gives attachment to all except—
(A) salpingopharyngeus
(B) thyropharyngeus
(C) stylopharyngeus
(D) palatopharyngeus

48. Muscles attached to oblique line of thyroid cartilage are all except -
(A) thyrohyoid
(B) sternothyroid
(C) middle constrictor
(D) inferior constrictor

49. True about cricoid cartilage is all except –
(A) paired cartilage of larynx
(B) narrow anterior & broad posterior arch
(C) situated at the level of C6 vertebra
(D) encircles lumen of larynx completely

50. All muscles elevate the larynx except-
(A) salpingopharyngeus
(B) sternothyroid
(C) stylopharyngeus
(D) palatopharyngeus

51. Muscle that opens the inlet of larynx is-
(A) aryepiglotticus
(B) oblique arytenoids
(C) thyroepiglotticus
(D) none of the above

52. Muscle that relax the vocal cord is-
(A) vocalis
(B) cricothyroids
(C) thyroarytenoids
(D) none of the above

53. Muscle that abducts the vocal cord is-
(A) transverse arytenoids
(B) lateral cricoarytenoids
(C) posterior cricoarytenoids
(D) none of the above

54. Muscle lying on external surface of larynx is-
(A) cricothyroid
(B) oblique arytenoid
(C) transverse arytenoid
(D) thyroarytenoids

55. Cricothyroid is supplied by-
(A) recurrent laryngeal nerve
(B) external laryngeal nerve
(C) glossopharyngeal nerve
(D) internal laryngeal nerve

56. Cartilage called as foundation stone of larynx-
(A) thyroid
(B) cricoid
(C) epiglottis
(D) none of the above

57. Safety muscle of larynx is-
(A) posterior cricoarytenoid
(B) cricothyroid
(C) transverse arytenoid
(D) none of the above

58. Commonest site of laryngeal cancer is-
(A) glottis region
(B) supra glottis region
(C) inlet of larynx
(D) all of the above

59. Modulator of voice is-
(A) vocalis
(B) posterior cricoarytenoid
(C) cricothyroid
(D) transverse arytenoid

60. Commonest type of cancer of larynx-
(A) squamous cell carcinoma
(B) adenocarcinoma
(C) mixed cell tumor
(D) none of the above

Answersheet

1. B, 2. A, 3. B, 4. C, 5. D, 6. D, 7. C, 8. D, 9. D, 10. D, 11. B, 12. C, 13. C, 14. B, 15. B, 16. B, 17. C, 18. C, 19. A, 20. D, 21. D, 22. B, 23. D, 24. D, 25. B, 26. D, 27. D, 28. B, 29. A, 30. D, 31. C, 32. C, 33. D, 34. B, 35. B, 36. B, 37. D, 38. C, 39. C, 40. C, 41. C, 42. B, 43. B, 44. B, 45. B, 46. B, 47. B, 48. C, 49. A, 50. B, 51. C, 52. C, 53. C, 54. A, 55. B, 56. B, 57. A, 58. A, 59. A, 60. A

Chapter 11

Orbit, Nose & Ear

1. Roof of the nose is formed by –
(A) cribriform plate of ethmoid
(B) nasal spine of frontal
(C) body of sphenoid
(D) all of the above

2. Smallest nasal concha is-
(A) superior nasal concha
(B) middle nasal concha
(C) inferior nasal concha
(D) all are equal

3. Largest nasal concha is-
(A) superior nasal concha
(B) middle nasal concha
(C) inferior nasal concha
(D) all are equal

4. Nasal concha which is a seprate bone is-
(A) superior nasal concha
(B) middle nasal concha
(C) inferior nasal concha
(D) all are part of ethmoid bone

5. Correct statement about nasal concha is-
(A) superior nasal concha is an independent bone
(B) middle nasal concha is part of sphenoid
(C) inferior nasal concha is seprate bone
(D) all nasal concha are part of ethmoid bone

6. Largest meatus is-
(A) superior meatus
(B) middle meatus
(C) inferior meatus
(D) all are equal

7. All are seen under middle meatus except-
(A) bulla ethmoidalis
(B) hiatus semilunaris
(C) Sphenoethmoidal recess
(D) infundibulum

8. Opening in superior meatus is-
(A) nasolacrimal duct
(B) anterior ethmoidal sinus
(C) posterior ethmoidal sinus
(D) middle ethmoidal sinus

9. Structures opening in middle meatus are-
(A) maxillary sinus
(B) frontal sinus
(C) middle & anterior ethmoidal sinuses
(D) all of the above

10. Sinus opening on bulla ethmoidalis-
(A) maxillary sinus
(B) frontal sinus
(C) anterior ethmoidal sinuses
(D) middle ethmoidal sinus

11. Sinus opening on hiatus semilunaris are -
(A) maxillary sinus
(B) frontal sinus
(C) anterior ethmoidal sinus
(D) all of the above

12. Nasolacrimal duct opens into-
(A) superior meatus of nose
(B) middle meatus of nose
(C) inferior meatus of nose
(D) superior most meatus of nose

13. Arteries supplying the nasal septum are all except –
(A) anterior ethmoidal branch of ophthalmic artery
(B) sphenopalatine branch of ascending pharyngeal artery artery
(C) septal branch of superior labial artery of facial artery
(D) sphenopalatine & greater palatine branch of maxillary artery

14. Arteries supplying the lateral wall of nose are –
(A) anterior ethmoidal branch of ophthalmic artery
(B) greater palatine & facial artery
(C) sphenopalatine branch of maxillary artery
(D) all of the above

15. Viens of the nasal cavity drain into-
(A) pterygoid venous plexus
(B) pharyngeal venous plexus
(C) facial vein
(D) all of the above

16. Lymphatic drainage of nose-
(A) submandibular & retromandibular lymph nodes
(B) retropharyngeal nodes & sublingual lymph nodes
(C) submandibular & retropharyngeal lymph nodes
(D) all of the above

17. Nerve supplying the nasal cavity are-
(A) olfactory nerve
(B) anterior ethmoidal nerve
(C) infraorbital nerve
(D) all of the above

18. Anterior group of sinuses include all except-
(A) frontal sinus
(B) maxillary sinus
(C) anterior & middle ethmoidal sinuses
(D) sphenoidal sinus

19. Anterior group of para nasal sinus drain into-
(A) superior meatus
(B) middle meatus
(C) inferior meatus
(D) any of above

20. True about maxillary air sinus is-
(A) first sinus to develop
(B) largest air sinus
(C) drains into hiatus semilunaris
(D) all of the above

21. Incorrect statement about hiatus semilunaris is-
(A) maxillary air sinus opens in anterior part
(B) frontal air sinus opens in anterior part
(C) anterior ethmoidal sinus opens in middle part
(D) maxillary air sinus opens in posterior part

22. Nasolacrimal duct lies in bony canal made up of all except-
(A) maxilla
(B) middle nasal concha
(C) lacrimal
(D) inferior nasal concha

23. True about relations of maxillary sinus is-
(A) infraorbital nerve & artery in roof
(B) anterior superior alveolar nerve in anterior wall
(C) posterior superior alveolar nerve & vessels in posterior wall
(D) all are true

24. True about canalis sinosus is-
(A) present in anterior wall of maxillary air sinus
(B) present in posterior wall of maxillary air sinus
(C) present in roof of maxillary air sinus
(D) present in floor of maxillary air sinus

25. Artery of nose bleeding is-
(A) septal branch of facial artery
(B) septal branch of sphenopalatine artery
(C) septal branch of anterior ethmoidal artery
(D) none of the above

26. Most commonly infected sinus is-
(A) frontal sinus
(B) maxillary sinus
(C) ethmoidal sinus
(D) sphenoidal sinus

27. Sinus which develops after birth-
(A) maxillary air sinus
(B) frontal air sinus
(C) sphenoidal air sinus
(D) ethmoidal air sinus

28. Lateral surface of pinna is supplied by-
(A) upper 2/3 by Auriculotemporal nerve
(B) lower 1/3 by great auricular nerve
(C) concha by auricular branch of vagus
(D) all of the above

29. Cranial surface of pinna is supplied by all except-
(A) upper 2/3 by lesser occipital nerve
(B) lower 1/3 by great auricular nerve
(C) Eminentia concha by auricular branch of vagus
(D) upper 2/3 by Auriculotemporal nerve

30. True about external auditory meatus is all except -
(A) 24 mm legth ,outer 1/3 cartilagenous & inner 2/3 bony
(B) isthmus is narrowest part at junction of bony & cartilage part
(C) isthmus is present at 20 mm deep in bony part
(D) in new born bony canal is not developed and represented by tympanic ring

31. Arterial supply to external acoustic meatus is from-
(A) anterior auricular artery branch of maxillary artery
(B) posterior auricular artery branch of external carotid artery
(C) deep auricular artery branch of maxillary artery
(D) all of the above

32. External auditory meatus develops from-
(A) an ectodermal derivative of 2nd pharyngeal cleft
(B) an endodermal derivative of 2nd pharyngeal cleft
(C) an endodermal derivative of 1st,2nd & 3rd pouches
(D) an ectodermal derivative of 1st pharyngeal cleft

33. Tympanic membrane is triple layered–
(A) outer cuticular layer of stratified epithelium
(B) middle fibrous layer & encloses handle of malleus
(C) inner layer is mucosal and covered by low columnar
(D) all are true

34. Tympanic membrane makes an angle with floor of external acoustic meatus-
(A) 35^0
(B) 45^0
(C) 55^0
(D) 65^0

35. Nerves supplying tympanic membrane–
(A) tympanic branch of glossopharyngeal nerve
(B) Auriculotemporal nerve
(C) auricular branch of vagus
(D) all of the above

36. Arteries supplying tympanic membrane –
(A) deep auricular artery – maxillary artery
(B) anterior tympanic artery – maxillary artery
(C) posterior tympanic artery – posterior auricular artery
(D) all of the above

37. Venous drainage of tympanic membrane –
(A) outer surface-external jugular vein
(B) inner surface-transverse sinus
(C) inner surface- pterygoid venous plexus
(D) all of the above

38. True about tympanic membrane is-
(A) outer cuticular layer-ectodermal in origin
(B) inner mucous layer-endodermal in origin
(C) middle layer-mesodermal in origin
(D) all of the above

39. Chorda tympani nerve is related to tympanic membrane-
(A) inner aspect of tympanic membrane in upper half on inner aspect
(B) crosses handle of malleus
(C) nerve is in between fibrous layer and mucosal layer
(D) all are true

40. Middle ear cavity contains-
(A) ear ossicles
(B) stapedius & tensor tympani
(C) chorda tympani nerve
(D) all of the above

41. Contents in epitympanum (attic) are all except-
(A) handle of malleus
(B) head of malleus
(C) body of incus
(D) short process of incus

42. Contents in mesotympanum are all except-
(A) head of malleus
(B) handle of malleus
(C) long process of incus
(D) stapes

43. Narrowest part of tympanic cavity is-
(A) epitympanum
(B) mesotympanum
(C) hypotympanum
(D) none of the above

44. Nerve piercing the floor of tympanic cavity is-
(A) chorda tympani nerve
(B) vagus nerve
(C) glossopharyngeal nerve
(D) facial nerve

45. Anterior wall of tympanic cavity is related to-
(A) tensor tympani muscle
(B) pharyngo tympanic tube
(C) internal carotid artery
(D) all of the above

46. Posterior wall of tympanic cavity is related to-
(A) stapedius muscle
(B) facial nerve
(C) chorda tympani nerve
(D) all of the above

47. Tympanic plexus is located on –
(A) lateral wall
(B) medial wall
(C) posterior wall
(D) roof of tympanic cavity

48. True about chorda tympani nerve is-
(A) lies between inner & middle layers of tympanic membrane
(B) runs lateral to long process of incus & medial to handle of malleus
(C) leaves through anterior canaliculus
(D) all of the above

49. Head of malleus articulates with body of incus-incudomalleolar joint -
(A) ball & socket variety
(B) saddle variety
(C) plain synovial joint
(D) hinge variety

50. Joint between incus & stapes-incudo-stapedial joint is-
(A) ball & socket variety
(B) saddle variety
(C) plain synovial joint
(D) hinge variety

51. Facial nerve in middle ear gives following branches except-
(A) chorda tympani nerve
(B) greater petrosal nerve
(C) lesser petrosal nerve
(D) nerve to stapedius muscle

52. Tympanic plexus is formed by all except-
(A) tympanic branch of glossopharyngeal nerve
(B) superior & inferior carotico-tympanic nerves
(C) branch from geniculate ganglion
(D) tympanic branch of vagus

53. Smallest skeletal muscle in the body-
(A) tensor tympani
(B) stapedius
(C) procerrus
(D) levator palpabre superioris

54. Fetus can hear sounds at-
(A) 16 week of IUL
(B) 20 week of IUL
(C) 24 week of IUL
(D) 28 week of IUL

55. Safest quadrant of tympanic membrane for myringotomy-
(A) anterior superior quadrant
(B) posterior inferior quadrant
(C) posterior superior quadrant
(D) anterior inferior quadrant

56. Smallest long bone of the body
(A) malleus
(B) incus
(C) stapes
(D) none of the above

57. Smallest bone of the body
(A) malleus
(B) incus
(C) stapes
(D) none of the above

58. Thinnest wall of orbit is-
(A) medial wall
(B) lateral wall
(C) roof
(D) floor

59. Strongest wall of orbit is-
(A) medial wall
(B) lateral wall
(C) roof
(D) floor

60. Medial wall of orbit is formed by-
(A) frontal & lacrimal process of maxilla
(B) body of sphenoid
(C) orbital plate of ethmoid
(D) all of the above

61. Floor of orbit is formed by-
(A) orbital surface of body of maxilla
(B) orbital surface of zygomatic bone
(C) orbital process of palatine bone
(D) all of the above

62. Levator palpebrae superioris is supplied by-
(A) occulomotor nerve
(B) trochleat nerve
(C) facial nerve
(D) abduscent nerve

63. Optic nerve is crossed by-
(A) superior opthlamic vein
(B) opthalmic artery
(C) nasocilliary nerves
(D) all of the above

64. All are supplied by inferior division of occulomotor except-
(A) superior rectus
(B) inferior rectus
(C) inferior oblique
(D) medial rectus

65. Smallest of three divisions of trigeminal nerve is-
(A) ophthalmic division
(B) maxillary division
(C) mandibular division
(D) all of the above

66. Branches of ophthalmic nerve are all except -
(A) lacrimal nerve
(B) frontal nerve
(C) infra orbital nerve
(D) nasociliary nerve

67. Smallest branch of opthalmic nerve is-
(A) lacrimal nerve
(B) frontal nerve
(C) nasociliary nerve
(D) all of the above

68. Largest branch of opthalmic nerve is-
(A) lacrimal nerve
(B) frontal nerve
(C) nasociliary nerve
(D) all of the above

69. About ophthalmic artery all are true except-
(A) branch of internal carotid artery
(B) arises within apex of cavernous sinus
(C) arises medial to anterior clenoid process
(D) enters orbit through optic canal inferolateral to optic nerve

70. Central artery of retina-
(A) first branch of ophthalmic artery
(B) arises within dural sheath
(C) supplies optic nerve & retina
(D) all of the above

71. Superior ophthalmic vein –
(A) passes through superior orbital fissure
(B) runs along with ophthalmic artery
(C) drains into cavernous venous sinus
(D) all of the above

72. Action of superior oblique is-
(A) elevation, abduction & intorsion
(B) elevation, adduction & intorsion
(C) depression, abduction & intorsion
(D) depression, abduction & extorsion

73. Action of inferior oblique is-
(A) elevation, abduction & intorsion
(B) elevation, abduction & extorsion
(C) elevation, adduction & intorsion
(D) depression, abduction & intorsion

74. Action of superior rectus is-
(A) elevation, abduction & intorsion
(B) elevation, adduction & intorsion
(C) elevation, adduction & extorsion
(D) depression, abduction & intorsion

75. Action of inferior rectus is-
(A) elevation, abduction & intorsion
(B) depression, adduction & extorsion
(C) elevation, adduction & extorsion
(D) depression, abduction & intorsion

76. True about eye ball is-
(A) outer coat sclera and cornea
(B) middle vascular coat is choroid,ciliary body & iris
(C) inner coat of retina
(D) all of the above

77. All structures in orbit lie inside the orbital periosteum except-
(A) infraorbital nerve
(B) zygomatic nerve
(C) infraorbital vessels
(D) all of the above

78. Uveal tract consists of-
(A) choroid
(B) ciliary body
(C) iris
(D) all of the above

79. Wrong statement about trochlear nerve is-
(A) longest intracranial course
(B) only cranial nerve arising from dorsal aspect of brain
(C) supplies ipsilateral superior oblique
(D) enters through superior orbital fissure

80. **Ocular muscle not arising from apex of the orbit-**
(A) superior rectus
(B) superior oblique
(C) inferior rectus
(D) inferior oblique

81. **Ligament of lookwood is seen in-**
(A) orbit
(B) pharynx
(C) larynx
(D) temporomandibular joint

82. **All are true for occulomotor nerve except-**
(A) have parasympathetic component
(B) supplies inferior oblique
(C) passes through inferior orbital fissure
(D) constriction of pupil

83. **Lamina cribrosa is a modification of-**
(A) choroid
(B) sclera
(C) retina
(D) nerve sheath of optic nerve

84. **Intortor of eye is-**
(A) inferior rectus
(B) superior rectus
(C) inferior oblique
(D) lateral rectus

85. **Actions of superior oblique are all except-**
(A) depression
(B) abduction
(C) extorsion
(D) intorsion

86. **Not a content of upper part of superior orbital fissure-**
(A) frontal nerve
(B) trochlear nerve
(C) occulomotor nerve
(D) lacrimal nerve

87. **Not passing through common tendinious ring of superior orbital fissure-**
(A) nasocillary nerve
(B) trochlear nerve
(C) occulomotor nerve
(D) abduscent nerve

88. **Ciliary ganglion is located-**
(A) apex of orbit between optic nerve & medial rectus
(B) apex of orbit between optic nerve & lateral rectus
(C) apex of orbit between optic nerve & inferior rectus
(D) none of the above

89. **Cornea is supplied by-**
(A) anterior ciliary arteries
(B) long ciliary arteries
(C) no arterial supply
(D) central artery of retina

90. **Maximum refraction by eye takes place at –**
(A) anterior surface of cornea
(B) posterior surface of retina
(C) aqueous humor
(D) none of the above

91. **Lymphatics from eye ball –**
(A) drain into pre auricular lymph nodes
(B) drain into parotid group of lymph nodes
(C) sub mental group of lymph nodes
(D) have no lymphatics

92. **Opening of maxillary sinus is in-**
(A) superior meatus
(B) middle meatus
(C) inferior meatus
(D) highest meatus

93. Nasolacrimal duct opens in-
(A) superior meatus
(B) middle meatus
(C) inferior meatus
(D) highest meatus

94. Mucous membrane of maxillary sinus is lined with-
(A) stratifed squamous epithelium
(B) stratifed columnar epithelium
(C) pseudostratifed cuboidal epithelium
(D) ciliated columnar epithelium

Answersheet

1. D, 2. A, 3. C, 4. C, 5. C, 6. C, 7. C, 8. C, 9. D, 10. D, 11. D, 12. C, 13. B, 14. D, 15. D, 16. C, 17. D, 18. D, 19. B, 20. D, 21. A, 22. B, 23. D, 24. A, 25. B, 26. B, 27. B, 28. D, 29. D, 30. B, 31. D, 32. D, 33. D, 34. C, 35. D, 36. D, 37. D, 38. D, 39. D, 40. D, 41. A, 42. A, 43. B, 44. C, 45. D, 46. D, 47. B, 48. D, 49. B, 50. A, 51. C, 52. D, 53. B, 54. B, 55. B, 56. A, 57. C, 58. A, 59. B, 60. D, 61. D, 62. A, 63. D, 64. A, 65. A, 66. C, 67. A, 68. B, 69. B, 70. D, 71. D, 72. C, 73. B, 74. B, 75. B, 76. D, 77. D, 78. D, 79. C, 80. D, 81. A, 82. C, 83. B, 84. B, 85. C, 86. C, 87. B, 88. B, 89. C, 90. A, 91. D, 92. B, 93. C, 94. D

Section - 2
Brain

Section - 3
Embryology

Section - 4
Histology

Chapter 1

General Neuroanatomy

1. Peripheral nervous system consists of all except-
(A) spinal cord
(B) ganglia
(C) cranial nerves
(D) spinal nerves

2. Homeostasis of body is maintained by-
(A) endocrine & reproductive system
(B) endocrine & nervous system
(C) nervous & immune system
(D) immune & reproductive system

3. False statement is-
(A) there are seven pairs of cervical spinal nerves
(B) there are twelve pairs of cranial nerves
(C) there are thirty one pairs of dorsal root ganglia
(D) all cranial nerves are not associated with ganglias

4. Correct statement is-
(A) all cranial nerves are attached to ventral surface of brain
(B) one cranial nerve is also attached to ventral aspect of spinal cord
(C) only one cranial nerve is attached to dorsal aspect of brain
(D) all cranial nerves are attached to dorsal aspect of brain

5. Nervous tissue consists of all except-
(A) neurons & their processes
(B) neuroglia
(C) connective tissue
(D) blood vessels

6. True about schwann cells is-
(A) present in peripheral nervous system only
(B) derived from neural crest
(C) help in regeneration of nerve fibers
(D) all of the above

7. All is true about astrocytes except-
(A) secrete growth stimulant
(B) cover brain surface & surface of neurons in ganglia
(C) form blood brain barrier
(D) are metabolic neurotransmitter

8. Neuroglial cells not present in CNS is-
(A) ependymal cell
(B) fibrous astrocytes
(C) oligodendrocytes
(D) satellite cells

9. Nerve cell unable to propogate impulse is-
(A) neuroglia
(B) golgi type-2 neurons
(C) interneurons
(D) motor neurons

10. True about oligodendrocytes is-
(A) only seen in CNS
(B) develop from neural crest
(C) produce mylin sheath in CNS
(D) all of the above

11. True about microglia is all except-
(A) phagocytic activity in CNS
(B) mesodermal in origin
(C) neral crest in origin
(D) highly active in degenerative disorders of CNS

12. Microglia is highly active in-
(A) multiple sclerosis
(B) alzheimer's disease
(C) parkinson's disease
(D) all of the above

13. Schwan's cells are-
(A) seen in PNS
(B) neural crest in origin
(C) produce myelin sheath and its regeneration
(D) all are true

14. Satellite cells –
(A) surround spinal & autonomic ganglion
(B) provide nutrition
(C) insulate and support the neurons in ganglion
(D) all of the above

15. True about nissl substance is all except-
(A) are aggregates of rough endoplasmic retinaculum
(B) dendrites contain and axon lack nissl granules
(C) are alkaline in nature
(D) are acidic in nature

16. Neurons seen in dorsal nerve root ganglion are-
(A) bipolar
(B) pseudounipolar / unipolar
(C) multipolar
(D) anaxonic

17. Bipolar neurons are seen in-
(A) spiral ganglion of vestibular nerve
(B) retina
(C) olfactory neuroepithelium
(D) all of the above

18. Pseudo unipolar neurons are seen in-
(A) mesencephalic nucleus of trigeminal nerve
(B) dorsal root ganglia of spinal nerves
(C) sensory ganglion of cranial nerves
(D) all of the above

19. Anaxonic neurons-
(A) do not have axons
(B) have only dendritic process
(C) seen amacrine cells of retina
(D) all of the above

20. False statement about Golgi type 1 neurons -
(A) have a single long axons
(B) seen in pyramidal tracts & spinal motor neurons
(C) seen in cerebellum
(D) purkinje cells

21. True about Golgi type 2 neurons –
(A) short axons
(B) inhibitory in nature
(C) seen in cerebellar cortex, stellate & granule cells
(D) all of the above

22. Most common cells producing tumors in brain is-
(A) schwann cells
(B) glial cells
(C) astrocytes
(D) microglial cells

23. Unmylinated nerve fibers are –
(A) covered by endoneurium
(B) covered by schwann cell sheath
(C) covered by both
(D) not covered

24. True about myelin sheath -
(A) made up of lipoprotein-myelin
(B) formed by Schwann cells in PNS
(C) formed by oligodendria in CNS
(D) all of the above

25. Demylelinating disorders are –
(A) multiple sclerosis
(B) guilian barre syndrome
(C) tay-sachs-disease
(D) all of the above

26. Heavy meals may be a cause of Demylelinating disease-
(A) mercury
(B) lead
(C) arsenic
(D) all of the above

27. Infection that may cvaus damage to myelin sheath –
(A) typhoid
(B) diptheria
(C) black water fever
(D) meningitis

28. Conduction velocity of nerve fibers –
(A) increases in cold climate
(B) increases in warm climate
(C) decreases in warm climate
(D) no effect of temperature

29. Features of Type A fibers –
(A) myelinated and large diameter
(B) motor neurons
(C) conduction velocity is more than 15-20 mtrs/sec
(D) all of the above

30. Features of Type C fibers –
(A) unmyelinated and small diameter
(B) carry pain and cold sensations
(C) conduction velocity is slow
(D) all of the above

Answer Sheet

1. A, 2. B, 3. A, 4. C, 5. C, 6. D, 7. B, 8. D, 9. A, 10. D, 11. C, 12. D, 13. D, 14. D, 15. C, 16. B, 17. D, 18. D, 19. D, 20. C, 21. D, 22. B, 23. B, 24. D, 25. D, 26. D, 27. B, 28. B, 29. D, 30. D

Chapter 2

Cranial Nerves

1. Cranial nerve not directly related to eye
   (A) 2nd cranial nerve
   (B) 3rd cranial nerve
   (C) 4th cranial nerve
   (D) 7th cranial nerve

2. Responsible for the movement of trazepius muscle
   (A) 9th cranial nerve
   (B) 10th cranial nerve
   (C) 11th cranial nerve
   (D) 12th cranial nerve

3. Sensations from anterior 2/3rd of tongue are carried by-
   (A) 12th cranial nerve
   (B) 9th cranial nerve
   (C) 7th cranial nerve
   (D) 10th cranial nerve

4. Nerve related to cardio-respiratory functions is-
   (A) 5th cranial nerve
   (B) 9th cranial nerve
   (C) 10th cranial nerve
   (D) 11thcranial nerve

5. Ptosis is due to –
   (A) 6th cranial nerve
   (B) 4th cranial nerve
   (C) 3rd cranial nerve
   (D) 2nd cranial nerve

6. Superior oblique muscle is supplied by-
   (A) 6th cranial nerve
   (B) 4th cranial nerve
   (C) 3rd cranial nerve
   (D) 7th cranial nerve

7. Not a feature of occulomotor palsy-
   (A) miosis
   (B) diffulcty in accomodation
   (C) superior gaze palsy
   (D) diplopia

8. Inferior oblique of eye is supplied by-
   (A) 3rd cranial nerve
   (B) 4TH cranial nerve
   (C) 6th cranial nerve
   (D) 7th cranial nerve

9. Occulomotor nerve supplies all except-
   (A) superior rectus
   (B) inferior oblique
   (C) lateral rectus
   (D) medial rectus

10. Disability in looking down and laterally is because of-
(A) occulomotor n
(B) trochlear n
(C) abduscent n
(D) ophthalmic n

11. Nerve passing through Meckel's cave is
(A) trochlear n
(B) trigeminal n
(C) abduscent n
(D) facial n

12. All are true about Trochlear n except-
(A) has longest intracranial course
(B) supplies ipsilateral superior oblique muscle
(C) arises from dorsal aspect of brain
(D) enters orbit through superior orbital fissure

13. All structures pass through superior orbital fissure except-
(A) occulomotor n
(B) ophthalmic n
(C) optic n
(D) trochlear n

14. Tensor tympani muscle is supplied by-
(A) maxillary n
(B) mandibular n
(C) glossopharyngeal n
(D) facial n

15. Tympanic plexus is formed by-
(A) mandibular n
(B) facial n
(C) glossopharyngeal n
(D) vagus n

16. Pinna is supplied by mainly-
(A) auriculo-temporal n
(B) auricular branch of vagus
(C) greater auricular n
(D) all of the above

17. External auditory meatus is supplied by-
(A) greater auricular n
(B) auriculo-temporal n
(C) facial n
(D) posterior auricular n

18. Pinna is supplied by all except-
(A) Auriculotemporal n
(B) Greater auricular n
(C) Vagus n
(D) Greater petrossal n

19. Alderman's nerve is
(A) auricular branch of glossopharyngeal n
(B) auricular branch of vagus n
(C) auricular branch of accessory cranial n
(D) auricular branch of facial n

20. Injury of 8th cranial n may lead to loss of-
(A) taste sensation
(B) touch sensation
(C) equilibrium sensation
(D) pressure sensation

21. Intrinsic muscles of tongue are supplied by-
(A) lingual n
(B) mandibular n
(C) hypoglossal n
(D) glossopharyngeal n

22. Pain of ulcers on the base of tongue are carried by-
(A) lingual n
(B) chorda tympani n
(C) glossopharyngeal n
(D) vagus n

23. Anterior 2/3rd of the tongue is supplied by-
(A) lingual n
(B) chorda tympani n
(C) glossopharyngeal n
(D) all of the above

24. All supply to anterior 2/3rd of tongue except
(A) lingual n
(B) vagus n
(C) glossopharyngeal n
(D) hypoglossal n

25. Posterior 1/3rd of the tongue is supplied by all except-
(A) glossopharyngeal n- general sensations
(B) glossopharyngeal n-taste sensations
(C) hypoglossal-motor
(D) lingual n-general sensations

26. Muscle supplied by glossopharyngeal n is-
(A) styloglossus
(B) stylopharyngeus
(C) stylohyoid
(D) salpingopharyngeus

27. Palate is supplied by all except-
(A) trigeminal n
(B) facial n
(C) glossopharyngeal n
(D) hypoglossal n

28. Pain in tonsillitis is carried by-
(A) lesser palatine n
(B) greater palatine n
(C) glossopharyngeal n
(D) lingual n

29. Eustchian tube is supplied by all except-
(A) glossopharyngeal n
(B) caratico-tympanic n
(C) accessory cranial n
(D) perygo-palatine ganglion

30. Internal laryngeal nerve supplies –
(A) cricothyroid muscle
(B) vocalis muscle
(C) mucosal membrane above vocal folds
(D) mucosal membrane below vocal folds

31. Damage to internal laryngeal nerve leads to-
(A) hoarseness of voice
(B) anaesthesia of larynx
(C) breathing diffulty
(D) aphonia

32. Mucosa of larynx is supplied by-
(A) superior laryngeal n
(B) external laryngeal n
(C) internal laryngeal
(D) recurrent laryngeal & external laryngeal n

33. Oral diaphragm is supplied by-
(A) inferior alveolar n
(B) nerve to mylohyoid
(C) lingual n
(D) massetric n

34. Parasympathetic secretomotor fibers to parotid gland travel through all except-
(A) tympanic plexus
(B) greater petrosal n
(C) otic ganglion
(D) Auriculotemporal n

35. Recurrent laryngeal nerve is in close association with-
(A) superior thyroid artery
(B) superior thyroid vein
(C) inferior thyroid artery
(D) superior thyroid vein

36. All are traversing through cavernous venous sinus except-
(A) occulomotor n
(B) trochlear n
(C) optic n
(D) abduscent n

37. All pass through lateral wall of cavernous venous sinus except-
(A) occulomotor n
(B) trochlear n
(C) abduscent n
(D) ophthalmic div of trigeminal n

38. Post trematic nerve of first branchial arch is-
(A) mandibular n
(B) chorda tympani n
(C) glossopharyngeal n
(D) facial n

39. Pre trematic nerve of second arch is-
(A) mandibular n
(B) jacobson'n
(C) vagus n
(D) facial n

40. Motor component of pharyngeal plexus is-
(A) trigeminal n
(B) hypoglossal n
(C) vagus n
(D) glossopharyngeal n

41. Sensory innervation of anterior 2/3rd of tongue is via-
(A) lingual branch of superior laryngeal n
(B) lingual branch of glossopharyngeal n
(C) lingual branch of trigeminal n
(D) lingual branch of vagus n

42. Larynx is supplied by –
(A) facial n
(B) glossopharyngeal n
(C) vagus n
(D) trigeminal n

43. Loss of sensations over parotid gland is due to injury of-
(A) facial n
(B) buccal n
(C) grater auricular n
(D) trigeminal n

44. All are supplied by facial nerve except-
(A) nasal glands
(B) parotid gland
(C) lacrimal gland
(D) submandibular gland

45. Cranial nerves present in posterior cranial fossa are-
(A) 3RD to 12TH
(B) 4TH to 12TH
(C) 5TH to 12TH
(D) 6TH to 12TH

46. Circumvallate papillae of the tongue present in anterior 2/3rd are supplied by-
(A) lingual n
(B) chorda tympani n
(C) glossopharyngeal n
(D) facial n

47. Vidian nerve is formed by-
(A) by joining greater superficial petrosal n & lesser petrosal n
(B) by joining deep petrosal n & greater superficial petrosal n
(C) by joining deep petrosal n & lesser superficial petrosal n
(D) all of the above

48. Which cranial nerve exits from pars nervosa of jugular foramen-
(A) glossoopharyngeal n
(B) vagus n
(C) cranial accessory n
(D) spinal accessory n

49. Nerve supplying to sublingual gland is-
(A) facial n
(B) auriculotemporal n
(C) inferior alveolar n
(D) glossopharyngeal n

50. Auriculotemporal nerve encircles which of the following artery-
(A) maxillary artery
(B) superficial temporal artery
(C) lingual artery
(D) middle meningeal artery

51. Infra orbital nerve is a branch from-
(A) optic n
(B) olfactory n
(C) maxillary n
(D) ophthalmic n

52. Injury of right mandibular nerve may result in-
(A) loss of taste sensations on anterior 2/3rd of right side of tongue
(B) loss of taste sensations on anterior 2/3rd of left side of tongue
(C) loss of general sensations on anterior 2/3rd of right side of tongue
(D) loss of taste sensations on posterior 1/3rd of right side of tongue

53. Nucleus ambiguus is related to following nerves
(A) 8th, 9th & 10th
(B) 9th, 10th &11th
(C) 10th, 11th & 12th
(D) 9th, 10th & 11th

54. All is true about inferior alveolar nerve except-
(A) branch of anterior division of mandibular nerve
(B) branch of posterior division of mandibular nerve
(C) enters mandibular canal
(D) comes out as mental nerve at mental foramen

55. Pharyngeal plexus of nervs is located on-
(A) superior constrictor of pharynx
(B) middle constrictor of pharynx
(C) inferior constrictor of pharynx
(D) all of the above

56. Pharyngeal plexus of nervs is formed by-
(A) glossopharyngeal nerve
(B) vagus nerve
(C) superior cervical sympathetic ganglion
(D) all othe above

57. Ansa cervicalis supplies all except-
(A) sternothyroid
(B) sternohyoid
(C) thyrohyoid
(D) omohyoid

58. Thyrohyoid is supplied by-
- (A) ansa cervicalis
- (B) nerve to thyrohyoid C1 from hypoglossal nerve
- (C) recurrent laryngeal nerve
- (D) internal laryngeal nerve

59. Posterior belly of digastric is supplied by-
- (A) mandibular nerve
- (B) facial nerve
- (C) great auricular nerve
- (D) occipital nerve

60. Anterior belly of digastric is supplied by-
- (A) mandibular nerve
- (B) facial nerve
- (C) great auricular nerve
- (D) occipital nerve

Answer Sheet

1. D, 2. C, 3. C, 4. C, 5. C, 6. B, 7. A, 8. A, 9. C, 10. B, 11. B, 12. B, 13. C, 14. B, 15. C, 16. D, 17. B, 18. D, 19. B, 20. C, 21. C, 22. C, 23. D, 24. B, 25. D, 26. B, 27. D, 28. C, 29. C, 30. C, 31. B, 32. C,

33. B, 34. B, 35. C, 36. C, 37. C, 38. A, 39. B, 40. C, 41. C, 42. C, 43. C, 44. B, 45. A, 46. C, 47. B, 48. A, 49. A, 50. D, 51. C, 52. C, 53. B, 54. A, 55. B, 56. D, 57. C, 58. B, 59. B, 60. A

Chapter 3

Spinal Cord

1. Spinal cord develops from-
   (A) proximal part of neural tube
   (B) distal part of neural tube
   (C) develops from whole of the neural tube
   (D) none

2. Most simple part of CNS is-
   (A) midbrain
   (B) pons
   (C) medulla
   (D) spinal cord

3. Diameter of spinal cord is minimum at–
   (A) cervical region
   (B) thoracic region
   (C) lumbar region
   (D) sacral region

4. Length of spinal cord is
   (A) 30 – 33 cms
   (B) 36 – 39 cms
   (C) 42 – 45 cms
   (D) 49 – 52 cms

5. Spinal cord starts at the vertebral level of -
   (A) C1
   (B) C1-C2
   (C) T1
   (D) none of the above

6. Lower border of spinal cord terminates at-
   (A) L1
   (B) L2
   (C) T12
   (D) S1

7. Cervical enlargement extends –
   (A) C3 to T1 spinal cord segment
   (B) C4 to T1 spinal cord segment
   (C) C4 to T2 spinal cord segment
   (D) C5 to T1 spinal cord segment

8. Lumbar enlargement extends –
   (A) L1 to S1 spinal cord segment
   (B) L1 to S2 spinal cord segment
   (C) L1 to S3 spinal cord segment
   (D) L2 to S4 spinal cord segment

9. Weight of spinal cord is-
   (A) 20 gms
   (B) 25 gms
   (C) 30 gms
   (D) 35 gms

10. Conus medullaris lies at the-
(A) T12 Vertebral level
(B) L1 Vertebral level
(C) L2 Vertebral level
(D) L3 Vertebral level

11. True about filum terminale is all except-
(A) extends from tip of conus medullaris to dorsum of 1st coccyx vertebrae
(B) made up of piamater, bluish in colour
(C) represents roots of rudimentary second & third sacral nerves
(D) surrounded by dura and arachnoid mater till S2

12. True about antero-median fissure of spinal cord is-
(A) 3 mm deep
(B) lodges anterior spinal artery
(C) reaches upto grey commisure
(D) all of the above

13. Wrong statement about spinal nerves is –
(A) cervical -7
(B) thoracic-12
(C) lumbar-5
(D) sacral -5

14. Grey matter of spinal cord consists of–
(A) motor neurons
(B) sensory neurons
(C) interneurons
(D) all of the above

15. Anterior grey columns of spinal cord consists of –
(A) cell bodies of alfa neurons
(B) cell bodies of gamma neurons
(C) Renshaw cells
(D) all of the above

16. Renshaw cells are -
(A) motor neurons
(B) sensory neurons
(C) interneurons
(D) all of the above

17. Lateral grey columns in spinal cord-
(A) contain preganglionic autonomic motor neurons
(B) seen at T1 to L2 & S2 toS4
(C) regulate smooth muscle, glandular & cardiac activites
(D) All of the above

18. Nuclei in anterior grey column are-
(A) medial group is seen throughout length of spinal cord
(B) central group is seen in cervical & lumbosacral region of spinal cord
(C) lateral group is seen in cervical & lumbar enlargement of cord
(D) all of the above

19. Central group of nuclei include all except-
(A) phrenic
(B) ventromedial nuclei
(C) spinal accessory nuclei
(D) lumbosacral nuclei

20. True about spinal accessory nucleus of spinal cord is all except-
(A) part of central group of nuclei
(B) present in cervical part of spinal cord
(C) present in cervical and lumbosacral part of spinal cord
(D) present in C1-C6 spinal segments

21. True about lumbosacral nuclei is all except-
(A) part of central group of nuclei
(B) present in lumbosacral part of spinal cord

(C) present in cervical part of spinal cord
(D) present in L2-S1 spinal segments

22. True about lateral group of nuclei in cervical enlargement is -
(A) ventrolateral nucleus supplies- shoulder & arm muscles
(B) dorsolateral nucleus supplies – forearm muscles
(C) retrodorsal nucleus supplies- hand muscles
(D) all of the above

23. True about lateral group of nuclei in lumbar enlargement is -
(A) ventrolateral nucleus supplies-hip & thigh muscles
(B) dorsolateral nucleus supplies –leg muscles
(C) retrodorsal nucleus supplies- foot muscles
(D) all of the above

24. True about substantia gelatinosa is-
(A) present near apex of posterior grey column in whole length of spinal cord
(B) consists of interneurons-modify sensory impulses
(C) continuous above as nucleus of spinal tract of trigeminal nerve
(D) all of the above

25. True about dorsal nucleus-Clarke's column is -
(A) thoracic nucleus extends from-C8 – L4
(B) present at the base of posterior grey column
(C) receives proprioceptive impulses from neuromuscular spindles & tendon end organs
(D) all of the above

26. True about laminar architecture of spinal cord is -
(A) lamina 10 occupy grey matter around central canal
(B) 1-6 occupy dorsal grey horn
(C) lamina 7 occupy intermediate grey mater, while 8 & 9 ventral grey horn
(D) all are true

27. Lamina 6 is absent in-
(A) C5 –T2
(B) T2 –L2
(C) T4 –L2
(D) none

28. True about clarke's column is-
(A) gives origin to dorsal spinocerebellar tract
(B) present in C8 –L3 and called nucleus dorsalis
(C) corresponds to lamina 5 &6
(D) all of the above

29. True about nucleus proprious is-
(A) gives origin to ventral spinothalamic tract
(B) present in entire length
(C) corresponds to lamina 3 & 4
(D) all of the above

30. White matter is maximum in –
(A) cervical part of spinal cord
(B) thoracic part of spinal cord
(C) lumbar part of spinal cord
(D) sacral part of spinal cord

31. At birth spinal cord extends upto-
(A) lower border of L1
(B) lower border of L3
(C) lower border of S1
(D) lower border of S3

Answer Sheet

1. B, 2. D, 3. B, 4. C, 5. A, 6. A, 7. C, 8. C, 9. C, 10. B, 11. C, 12. D, 13. A, 14. D, 15. D, 16. C, 17. D, 18. D, 19. B, 20. C, 21. C, 22. D, 23. D, 24. D, 25. D, 26. D, 27. D, 28. D, 29. D, 30. A, 31. B

Chapter 4

Medulla

1. Medulla oblongata shows –
   (A) anterior median fissure
   (B) posterior median fissure
   (C) both anterior and posterior median fissure
   (D) anterior median fissure and posterior median septum

2. Length of medulla is-
   (A) 1.3 cms
   (B) 2 cms
   (C) 3 cms
   (D) 4cms

3. Width (transverse diameter) of medulla is-
   (A) 1.3 cms
   (B) 2 cms
   (C) 3 cms
   (D) 4cms

4. Thickness (antero-posterior diameter) of medulla is-
   (A) 1.3 cms
   (B) 2 cms
   (C) 3 cms
   (D) 4cms

5. Closed part of medulla is-
   (A) upper 1/3 of medulla
   (B) lower 1/3 of medulla
   (C) upper 1/2 of medulla
   (D) lower 1/2 of medulla

6. Open part of medulla is-
   (A) upper 1/3 of medulla
   (B) lower 1/3 of medulla
   (C) upper 1/2 of medulla
   (D) lower 1/2 of medulla

7. Foramen caecum is seen in medulla –
   (A) anterior median fissure
   (B) posteromedian sulcus
   (C) not seen in medulla
   (D) both in antero and posteromedian fissures

8. Hypoglossal nerve is attached to medulla at –
   (A) antero-median sulcus
   (B) anterolateral sulcus
   (C) posterolateral sulcus
   (D) posteromedian sulcus

9. Glossopharyngeal nerve is attached to medulla at –
   (A) antero-median sulcus
   (B) anterolateral sulcus
   (C) posterolateral sulcus
   (D) posteromedian sulcus

10. Vagus nerve is attached to medulla at–
(A) antero-median sulcus
(B) anterolateral sulcus
(C) posterolateral sulcus
(D) posteromedian sulcus

11. Accessory nerve is attached to medulla at –
(A) antero-median sulcus
(B) anterolateral sulcus
(C) posterolateral sulcus
(D) posteromedian sulcus

12. All nerves are attached to posterolateral sulcus of medulla except –
(A) glossopharyngeal nerve
(B) vagus nerve
(C) accessory nerve
(D) hypoglossal nerve

13. Cranial nerve emerging at ponto-medullary junction just above to pyramid is-
(A) facial nerve
(B) abducent nerve
(C) trigeminal nerve
(D) vestibulocochlear nerve

14. Cranial nerve emerging at ponto-medullary junction just above to olive is-
(A) facial nerve
(B) abducent nerve
(C) trigeminal nerve
(D) vestibulocochlear nerve

15. Supra spinal nucleus seen in the lower part of medulla give rise to-
(A) glossopharyngeal nerve
(B) vagus nerve
(C) 1st cervical nerve
(D) accessory spinal nerve

16. Supra spinal nucleus seen in the lower part of medulla is contiguous with -
(A) glossopharyngeal nerve nucleus
(B) vagus nerve nucleus
(C) hypoglossal nucleus
(D) accessory spinal nerve nucleus

17. Spinal nucleus in medulla oblongata –
(A) give rise to accessory nerve
(B) continuous with upper 5 cervical spinal segments
(C) merges with nucleus ambiguus
(D) all of the above

18. Upwards extension of dorsal horn of spinal cord in medulla is-
(A) substantia gelatinosa
(B) supraspinal nucleus
(C) nucleus gracilis
(D) nucleus cuneatus

19. Internal arcuate fibres are-
(A) first order neurons
(B) second order neurons
(C) third order neurons
(D) none of the above

20. Internal arcuate fibres arise from-
(A) first order neurons from nucleus gracilis
(B) second order neurons from nucleus gracilis & cuneatus
(C) second order neurons from nucleus gracilis, cuneate & accessory cuneate nucleus
(D) none of the above

21. Posterior external arcuate fibres arise from-
(A) first order neurons from nucleus gracilis
(B) second order neurons from nucleus gracilis & cuneatus
(C) second order neurons from accessory cuneate nucleus
(D) second order neurons from cuneate & accessory cuneate nucleus

22. Posterior external arcuate fibres –
(A) ipsilateral and uncrossed
(B) arise from accessory cuneate nucleus
(C) reach cerebellum through inferior cerebellar peduncle
(D) all of the above

23. Posterior external arcuate fibres –
(A) carry impulses from upper limbs
(B) carry proprioceptive impulses
(C) forms Cuneo cerebellar tract
(D) all of the above

24. Nucleus tractus solitarious receives impulses from all except-
(A) facial nerve
(B) glossopharyngeal nerve
(C) vagus nerve
(D) hypoglossal

25. Arcuate nuclei in medulla are –
(A) displaced pontine nuclei
(B) form anterior external arcuate fibres
(C) placed anterior to pyramids at olivary nuclei
(D) all of the above

26. Retro facial nucleus is seen in-
(A) medulla
(B) pons
(C) mid brain
(D) none of the above

27. Nuclei present in central grey matter around central canal in closed part of medulla are all except-
(A) hypoglossal nucleus
(B) nucleus ambiguus
(C) nucleus of tractus solitarious
(D) dorsal nucleus of vagus

28. Nucleus not present in central grey matter around central canal in closed part of medulla is -
(A) hypoglossal nucleus
(B) nucleus ambiguus
(C) nucleus of tractus solitarious
(D) dorsal nucleus of vagus

29. Fasciculus gracilis & fasciculus gracilis are carrying –
(A) pain & temperature sensations
(B) proprioceptive sensation
(C) touch & pressure sensations
(D) all of the above

30. Fasciculus gracilis & fasciculus gracilis in medulla are having –
(A) first order of neurons
(B) second order of neurones
(C) third order of neurons
(D) all of the above

31. Fasciculus gracilis & fasciculus gracilis are carrying –
(A) pain & temperature sensations
(B) proprioceptive sensation
(C) touch & pressure sensations
(D) all of the above

32. Nucleus gracilis in medulla are having –
(A) first order of neurons
(B) second order of neurones
(C) third order of neurons
(D) all of the above

33. Medial longitudinal bundle is formed by –
(A) anterior external arcuate fibres
(B) internal arcuate fibres
(C) posterior external arcuate fibres
(D) none of the above

34. Medial lemniscus is formed by –
(A) anterior external arcuate fibres
(B) internal arcuate fibres
(C) posterior external arcuate fibres
(D) none of the above

35. Medial longitudinal bundle is formed by ascending and descending fibres from –
(A) III Nerve
(B) IV Nerve
(C) VII Nerve
(D) all of the above

36. Which arcuate fibres are not crossing to opposite side in medulla-
(A) anterior external arcuate fibres
(B) internal arcuate fibres
(C) posterior external arcuate fibres
(D) all of the above cross to opposite side

37. Striae medullaris are fibres run over the floor of fourth ventricle arise from-
(A) nucleus gracilis & cuneate
(B) accessory cuneate nucleus
(C) arcuate nucleus
(D) nucleus of tractus solitarious

38. Nucleus present in reticular formation at closed part of medulla is –
(A) dorsal nucleus of vagus
(B) nucleus ambiguus
(C) hypoglossal nucleus
(D) nucleus tractus solitarious

39. Nuclei present in the floor of fourth ventricle in open part of medulla are all except –
(A) vestibular nuclei
(B) vagus nucleus
(C) ambiguus nucleus
(D) hypoglossal nucleus

40. Medial medullary syndrome is due to occlusion of-
(A) anterior spinal artery
(B) posterior inferior cerebellar artery
(C) basilar artery
(D) all of the above

41. Lateral medullary syndrome is due to occlusion of-
(A) anterior spinal artery
(B) posterior inferior cerebellar artery
(C) basilar artery
(D) all of the above

42. Medulla is supplied by-
(A) anterior spinal artery
(B) posterior spinal artery
(C) posterior inferior cerebellar artery
(D) all of the above

43. Areas damaged in medial medullary syndrome are all except-
(A) hypoglossal nucleus
(B) nucleus ambiguus
(C) medial lemniscus
(D) pyramids

44. Areas damaged in lateral medullary syndrome are all except-
(A) lateral spinothalamic tract
(B) medial lemniscus
(C) vestibular nuclei
(D) nucleus ambiguus

45. Dysphagia is a typical feature of –
(A) medial medullary syndrome
(B) lateral syndrome
(C) both A & B
(D) none of the above

46. Dysphagia is a typical feature of –
(A) medial medullary syndrome
(B) lateral syndrome
(C) both A & B
(D) none of the above

47. Crossed or alternating paralysis is a typical feature of-
(A) medial medullary syndrome
(B) lateral syndrome
(C) both A & B
(D) none of the above

48. Lateral spinothalamic tract is typically involved in-
(A) medial medullary syndrome
(B) lateral medullary syndrome
(C) both A & B
(D) none of the above

49. Wallenberg's syndrome is due to occlusion of the –
(A) anterior spinal artery
(B) posterior spinal artery
(C) posterior inferior cerebellar artery
(D) none of the above

50. Nucleus not seen in medulla is-
(A) dorsal nucleus of vagus
(B) superior salivatory nucleus
(C) inferior salivatory nucleus
(D) nucleus of tractus solitarious

Answer Sheet

1. C, 2. C, 3. B, 4. A, 5. D, 6. C, 7. A, 8. B, 9. C, 10. C, 11. C, 12. D, 13. B, 14. A, 15. C, 16. C, 17. D, 18. A, 19. B, 20. B, 21. C, 22. D, 23. D, 24. D, 25. D, 26. A, 27. B, 28. B, 29. B, 30. A, 31. B, 32. B, 33. D, 34. B, 35. D, 36. C, 37. C, 38. B, 39. C, 40. A. 41. B, 42. D, 43. B, 44. B, 45. B, 46. B, 47. A, 48. B, 49. C, 50. B.

Chapter 5

Pons

1. Cranial nerve nucleuses of following nerves are seen at pons –
   (A) trigeminal nerve
   (B) abducent nerve
   (C) facial nerve
   (D) all of the above
2. Cranial nerve nucleuses of following nerves are seen at upper level of pons–
   (A) trigeminal nerve
   (B) abducent nerve
   (C) facial nerve
   (D) all of the above
3. Cranial nerve nucleuses of following nerves are seen at lower level of pons–
   (A) trigeminal nerve
   (B) abducent nerve
   (C) facial nerve
   (D) abducent and facial both
4. Nucleus seen at pons is/are –
   (A) superior olivary nucleus
   (B) inferior olivary nucleus
   (C) accessory olivary nucleus
   (D) all of the above
5. Facial colliculus is seen at–
   (A) upper level of pons
   (B) lower level of pons
   (C) ponto-medullary junction
   (D) all of the above
6. Nerve directly attached to pons is-
   (A) facial nerve
   (B) abducent nerve
   (C) trigeminal nerve
   (D) all of the above
7. Nerve attached to pontomedullary junction is/are-
   (A) facial nerve
   (B) abducent nerve
   (C) vestibulochochlear nerve
   (D) all of the above
8. Nerve attached most lateral at pontomedullary junction is -
   (A) facial nerve
   (B) abducent nerve
   (C) vestibulocochlear nerve
   (D) all of the above
9. Nerve attached most medial at pontomedullary junction is -
   (A) facial nerve
   (B) abducent nerve
   (C) vestibulocochlear nerve
   (D) all of the above

10. Nerve attached at pontomedullary junction above pyramid is -
(A) facial nerve
(B) abducent nerve
(C) trigeminal nerve
(D) vestibulocochlear nerve

11. Nerve attachment at ponto medullary junction from medial to lateral are-
(A) facial n, abducent n & vestibulocochlear n
(B) facial n, vestibulocochlear n & abducent n
(C) abducent n, vestibulocochlear n & facial n
(D) abducent n, facial n & vestibulocochlear n

12. Nerve attachment at ponto medullary junction from lateral to medial are-
(A) facial n, abducent n & vestibulocochlear n
(B) vestibulocochlear n, abducent n & facial n
(C) vestibulocochlear n, facial n & abducent nerve
(D) abducent n, facial n & vestibulocochlear n

13. Nucleus seen at pons are all except –
(A) superior salivatory nucleus
(B) special lacrimatory nucleus
(C) nucleus of tractus solitarious
(D) inferior salivatory nucleus

14. Nucleus of tractus solitarious is related to –
(A) facial nerve
(B) glossopharyngeal nerve
(C) vagus nerve
(D) all of the above

15. Trapezoid body is a part of –
(A) visual pathway
(B) auditory pathway
(C) taste pathway
(D) none of the above

16. Trapezoid body is a part of –
(A) medial lemniscus
(B) lateral lemniscus
(C) medial longitudinal bundle
(D) spinal lemniscus

17. Superior salivatory nucleus controls secretion from all except-
(A) submandibular gland
(B) parotid gland
(C) sublingual gland
(D) lacrimal gland

18. Trigeminal nerve is attached to pons by two roots true is –
(A) medial sensory large & lateral motor small root
(B) medial motor large & lateral sensory small root
(C) medial motor small & lateral sensory large root
(D) medial sensory small & lateral motor large root

19. All of the following nucleuses of trigeminal nerve are seen at pons except -
(A) motor nucleus
(B) spinal nucleus
(C) mesencephalic nucleus
(D) sensory nucleus

20. Haemorrhage in pons will lead to –
(A) internal squint
(B) external squint
(C) dilatation of pupil
(D) ptosis

21. Millard Gubler syndrome is due to the involvement of –
(A) mid brain
(B) pons
(C) medulla
(D) spinal cord

22. Characteristic features of Millard Gubler syndrome are –
(A) ipsilateral internal squint
(B) ipsilateral facial palsy
(C) contralateral hemiplegia
(D) all of the above

23. Areas of pons involved in the Millard Gubler syndrome are –
(A) abducent nerve
(B) facial nerve
(C) corticospinal fibres
(D) all of the above

24. Pons is having following lemniscuses –
(A) medial lemniscus
(B) lateral lemniscus
(C) trigeminal lemniscus
(D) all of the above

25. Pons is having following lemniscuses –
(A) medial lemniscus
(B) lateral lemniscus
(C) spinal lemniscus
(D) all of the above

26. Lemniscuses present at pons are organized from medial to lateral as-
(A) medial, lateral, trigeminal & spinal lemniscus
(B) lateral, medial, spinal & trigeminal lemniscus
(C) spinal, trigeminal, medial & lateral lemniscus
(D) medial, trigeminal, spinal & lateral lemniscus

27. Spinal lemniscus carries sensations of–
(A) visual
(B) auditory
(C) touch, pressure & temperature
(D) taste

28. Pin point pupil in the case of pontine haemorrhage happens due to involvement of –
(A) abducent nerve
(B) reticular formation
(C) corticonuclear fibres
(D) trapezoid body

29. Deep sleep and coma in the case of pontine haemorrhage happens due to involvement of –
(A) abducent nerve
(B) reticular formation
(C) corticonuclear fibres
(D) trapezoid body

30. Nerves intermedius lies in between –
(A) abducent medially & auditory laterally
(B) facial medially & abducent laterally
(C) facial medially & auditory laterally
(D) auditory medially & facial laterally

31. Largest part of brain stem is –
(A) midbrain
(B) pons
(C) medulla
(D) all are equal

32. Smallest part of brain stem is –
(A) midbrain
(B) pons
(C) medulla
(D) all are equal

33. Middle cerebellar peduncle is –
(A) smallest cerebellar peduncle
(B) largest cerebellar peduncle
(C) motor in function
(D) none of the above

34. Facial colliculus is seen at –
(A) midbrain
(B) upper level of pons
(C) lower level of pons
(D) medulla

35. All of the following nerves are attached at pontomedullary junction except –
(A) trigeminal nerve
(B) abducent nerve
(C) facial nerve
(D) vestibulocochlear nerve

36. Nerve attached at pontomedullary junction above pyramid is –
(A) trigeminal nerve
(B) abducent nerve
(C) facial nerve
(D) vestibulocochlear nerve

37. Nerve attached at pontomedullary junction above olive is/are –
(A) trigeminal nerve
(B) abducent nerve & facial nerve
(C) facial nerve & vestibulocochlear nerve
(D) vestibulocochlear nerve

38. Floor of the fourth ventricle in relation to pons has following areas –
(A) facial triangle
(B) vestibular area
(C) vagal area
(D) facial and vestibular areas

39. Floor of the fourth ventricle in relation to medulla has following areas –
(A) hypoglossal area
(B) vestibular area
(C) vagal area
(D) all of the above

40. Nucleus seen at pons is –
(A) inferior olivary nucleus
(B) medial accessory olivary nucleus
(C) superior olivary nucleus
(D) dorsal accessory olivary nucleus

41. Olivary nucleus associated with trapezoid body is-
(A) inferior olivary nucleus
(B) medial accessory olivary nucleus
(C) superior olivary nucleus
(D) dorsal accessory olivary nucleus

42. All of the following nuclei are part of superior olivary nuclear complex except –
(A) lateral sup olivary nu
(B) medial sup olivary nu
(C) retro olivary nucleus
(D) medial accessory olivary nucleus

43. All are seen in Raymond's syndrome –
(A) hemiplegia opposite side
(B) medial squint on same side
(C) ipsilateral facial palsy
(D) both A & B

44. Features of Foville's syndrome are
(A) ipsilateral squint
(B) ipsilateral facial palsy
(C) hemiparesis for brief duration on opposite side
(D) All of the above

Answer Sheet

1. D, 2. A, 3. D, 4. A, 5. A, 6. C, 7. D, 8. C, 9. B, 10. B, 11. D, 12. C, 13. D, 14. D, 15. B, 16. B, 17. B, 18. C, 19. C, 20. A, 21. B, 22. D, 23. 24. D, 25. D, 26. D, 27. C, 28. B, 29. B, 30. C, 31. B, 32. A, 33. B, 34. C, 35. A, 36. B, 37. C, 38. D, 39. D, 40. C, 41. C, 42. D, 43. D, 44. D.

Chapter 6

Midbrain

1. Midbrain contains following -
   (A) 3rd cranial nerve nucleus
   (B) 4th cranial nerve nucleus
   (C) cerebral aqueduct
   (D) all of the above
2. Superior colliculus are centre for-
   (A) auditory reflexes
   (B) visual reflexes
   (C) taste sensations
   (D) audio-visual reflexes
3. Inferior colliculus are centre for-
   (A) visual reflexes
   (B) auditory reflexes
   (C) balancing reflexes
   (D) audio-visual reflexes
4. Ventral part of midbrain-
   (A) two crus cerebri
   (B) interpeduncular fossa between them
   (C) posterior perforated substance in fossa
   (D) all are true
5. Interpeduncular fossa contains all except-
   (A) anterior perforated substance
   (B) mammillary bodies
   (C) posterior perforated substance
   (D) central branches of posterior cerebral artery
6. Crus cerebri is crossed transversely by all except-
   (A) optic tract
   (B) posterior cerebral artery
   (C) inferior cerebellar artery
   (D) superior cerebellar artery
7. On each side laterally crus cerebri is related to all except-
   (A) parahippocampal gyrus
   (B) lateral sulcus
   (C) oculomotor nerve
   (D) trochlear nerve
8. Cranial nerve arising from medial side of crus cerebri is-
   (A) optic nerve
   (B) olfactory nerve
   (C) oculomotor nerve
   (D) trochlear nerve
9. Cranial nerve arising from lateral side of crus cerebri is-
   (A) optic nerve
   (B) olfactory nerve
   (C) oculomotor nerve
   (D) trochlear nerve

10. Corpora quadrigemina is on the dorsal surface of midbrain-
(A) superior and inferior coliculi are seprated by cruciform sulcus
(B) superior coliculus is for visual reflexes
(C) inferior coliculus is for auditory reflexes
(D) all of the above

11. Trochlear nerve-
(A) originates from the dorsal aspect of brain
(B) runs across lateral aspect of crus cerebri
(C) runs between superior cerebellar and posterior cerebral arteries
(D) all are true

12. Brachium of superior colliculus-
(A) bands of white fibers
(B) connects optic tract & lateral geniculate body
(C) conveys visual impulses
(D) all are true

13. Brachium of inferior colliculus-
(A) bands of white fibers
(B) connects the inferior colliculus & medial geniculate body
(C) conveys auditory impulses
(D) all are true

14. All are parts of cerebral peduncle except-
(A) tectum
(B) tegmentum
(C) substantia nigra
(D) crus cerebri

15. Corticonuclear & corticospinal fibers are seen in –
(A) lateral 1/3rd of crus cerebri
(B) medial 1/3rd of crus cerebri
(C) middle 3/5th of crus cerebri
(D) lateral 2/3rd of crus cerebri

16. Corticopontine fibers from temporal, occipital & parietal lobes are seen in –
(A) lateral 1/5th of crus cerebri
(B) medial 1/3rd of crus cerebri
(C) middle 3/5th of crus cerebri
(D) lateral 2/3rd of crus cerebri

17. Corticopontine fibers from frontal lobe are seen in –
(A) medial 1/5th of crus cerebri
(B) medial 1/3rd of crus cerebri
(C) middle 3/5th of crus cerebri
(D) lateral 2/3rd of crus cerebri

18. Corticopontocerebellar pathway is part of-
(A) pyramidal system
(B) extrapyramidal system
(C) ascending system
(D) all of the above

19. True about substantia nigra is-
(A) band of dark grey matter
(B) extends throughout length of midbrain
(C) present in cerebral peduncle dorsal to crus cerebri
(D) all of the above

20. True about substantia nigra is-
(A) band of dark grey matter
(B) extends throughout length of midbrain
(C) present in cerebral peduncle dorsal to crus cerebri
(D) all of the above

21. True about substantia nigra is-
(A) pigmented nerve cells
(B) extends throughout length of midbrain
(C) iron & melanin pigment
(D) all of the above

22. **Substance P is seen in -**
(A) dorsal compact part of sustantia nigra
(B) ventral reticular part of substantia nigra
(C) both
(D) none

23. **Neurotansmiters present in reticular part of substantia nigra is-**
(A) GABA- gamma-amino-buteryic acid
(B) ENK-enkephalin
(C) 5-HT-serotonin
(D) all of the above

24. **Neurons of compact part of substantia nigra contain-**
(A) dopamine
(B) GABA
(C) 5-HT
(D) all of the above

25. **Lower level of midbrain at inferior colliculus contains all except-**
(A) trochlear nucleus
(B) mesencephalic nucleus
(C) locus coeruleus
(D) all of the above

26. **All are true about mesencephalic nucleus of trigeminal nerve except-**
(A) sensory nucleus
(B) contains unipolar neurons
(C) contains bipolar neurons
(D) receives proprioceptive sensations from face

27. **Lateral lemniscus ends in-**
(A) superior colliculus
(B) inferior colliclus
(C) collicular quadrigemina
(D) both superior & inferior colliculus

28. **True about inferior colliculus is all except-**
(A) large nucleus of auditory pathway
(B) afferent from lateral lemniscus
(C) efferents to lateral geniculate body
(D) efferents to medial geniculate body

29. **All are true about Edinger Westphal nucleus except-**
(A) visceral motor nucleus at inferior colliculus
(B) preganglionic parasympathetic fibers reach ciliary ganglion
(C) supplies ciliary muscle
(D) supplies constrictor pupillae muscle of iris

30. **Red nucleus-**
(A) seen at upper level of midbrain
(B) contains copper rich pigment
(C) part of extrapyramidal system
(D) motor nucleus and controls posture & muscle tone

31. **Lemniscus not seen at superior colliculus is-**
(A) medial lemniscus
(B) lateral lemniscus
(C) trigeminal lemniscus
(D) spinal lemniscus

32. **Superior colliculus is made up of-**
(A) five alternate layers of white and grey matter
(B) seven alternate layers of white and grey matter
(C) three alternate layers of white and grey matter
(D) none of the above

33. Zonal layer of superior colliculus receives-
(A) fibers from retina
(B) fibers from occipital cortex
(C) fibers from retina & occipital cortex both
(D) none of the above

34. Optic layer of superior colliculus receives-
(A) fibers from visual cortex area 17, 18 & 19
(B) fibers from retina
(C) fibers from retina & occipital cortex both
(D) none of the above

35. True about pretectal nucleus is all except-
(A) located at junction of midbrain & diencephalon
(B) receives afferent from both retina
(C) send efferent to Edinger Westphal nucleus of same side
(D) send efferent to Edinger Westphal nucleus of same side as well as to opposite

36. True about medial longitudinal bundle is all except-
(A) fibers from right and left vestibular nuclei are main constituents
(B) connects 3rd, 4th, 6th & 11th cranial nerves
(C) fibers arising from nucleus of medial lemniscus
(D) fibers arising from nucleus of lateral lemniscus

37. Weber's syndrome is due to occlusion of-
(A) anterior cerebral artery
(B) posterior cerebral artery
(C) middle cerebral artery
(D) posterior inferior cerebellar artery

38. In Weber's syndrome involved structures are-
(A) occulomotor nerve & corticospinal tracts
(B) occulomotor n, trochlear n & corticospinal tracts
(C) occulomotor n, Edinger Westphal nucleus & corticospinal tracts
(D) occulomotor n, Edinger Westphal nucleus, trochlear n & corticospinal tracts

39. Observations in Weber's syndrome are all except-
(A) dilatation of pupil on ipsilateral side
(B) drooping of eyelid & medial squint
(C) hemiparesis on contralateral side
(D) drooping of eyelid & lateral squint

40. In Benedict's syndrome involved structures are all except-
(A) corticospinal tracts
(B) occulomotor nucleus
(C) red nucleus
(D) trochlear nucleus

41. Observations in Benedict's syndrome are all except-
(A) dilatation of pupil on ipsilateral side
(B) drooping of eyelid & medial squint
(C) hemiparesis on contralateral side
(D) cerebellar tremors

42. Cranial nerve that takes origin from dorsal surface of brainstem is-
(A) occulomotor nerve
(B) trochlear nerve
(C) accessory nerve
(D) vagus nerve

Answer Sheet

1. D, 2. B , 3. B, 4. D, 5. A, 6. C, 7. C, 8. C, 9. D, 10. D, 11. D, 12. D, 13. D, 14. A, 15. C, 16. A, 17. A, 18. B, 19. D, 20. D, 21. D, 22. C, 23. D, 24. A, 25. D, 26. C, 27. B, 28. C, 29. A, 30. B, 31. B, 32. B, 33. B, 34. B, 35. C, 36. C, 37. B, 38. C, 39. B, 40. D, 41. B, 42. B

Chapter 7

Cerebellum

1. Hind brain consists of-
(A) medulla & pons
(B) pons, midbrain & cerebellum
(C) medulla, pons & cerebellum
(D) medulla, pons, midbrain & cerebellum

2. True about cerebellum is all except –
(A) motor activity without any conscious awareness
(B) contralateral control of the body
(C) ipsilateral control of the body
(D) maintenance of posture and balance

3. Primary fissure is present on-
(A) superior surface of cerebellum
(B) inferior surface of cerebellum
(C) between superior & inferior surface of cerebellum
(D) none of the above

4. Primary fissure seprates-
(A) anterior lobe & posterior (middle) lobe
(B) posterior & inferior lobe
(C) posterior & flocculonodular lobe
(D) none of the above

5. Archicerebellum is oldest and consists of all except-
(A) lingula
(B) nodule
(C) tonsil
(D) flocculus

6. Archicerebellum is-
(A) vestibular in connection
(B) flocculonodular lobe is main part
(C) responsible for maintenance of posture and balance
(D) all of the above

7. Paleocerebellum is-
(A) spinal in connection & regulates muscle tone
(B) ala, quadrangular lobe, culmen & central lobule of anterior lobe
(C) pyramid & uvula of posterior lobe
(D) all of the above

8. Neocerebellum is-
(A) most recent & cerebral in connection
(B) consists of posterior lobe except uvula & pyramid
(C) co-ordination of voluntary functions
(D) all of the above

9. All are true about cerebellum except-
(A) depends on termination of purkinje cell axonal termination on cerebellar nuclei
(B) four sagittal zones
(C) three sagittal zones
(D) lateral zone is largest

10. Three sagittal zones of cerebellum on functional basis are all except-
(A) vermal zone
(B) paravermal zone
(C) medial zone
(D) lateral zone

11. True about vermal zone is all except-
(A) dentate in connection
(B) unpaired midline portion of cerebellum
(C) controls posture, muscle tone & equilibrium
(D) fastigial in connection

12. True about para-vermal zone is all except-
(A) dentate in connection
(B) lateral to vermal zone of cerebellum
(C) controls muscle tone
(D) emboliformis & globose in connection

13. True about lateral zone is all except-
(A) controls muscle tone
(B) largest zone of cerebellum
(C) co-ordinates motor activities
(D) dentate in connection

14. Vestibulocerebellum is-
(A) floculonodular lobe
(B) lateral zone
(C) anterior lobe
(D) none of the above

15. Spinocerebellum consists of –
(A) vermal zone
(B) paravermal zone
(C) lateral zone
(D) A+B both

16. Cerebellar cortex is made up of all except-
(A) molecular layer
(B) purkinje layer
(C) pyramidal layer
(D) granular layer

17. True about molecular layer of cerebellum is -
(A) superficial layer just covered by piamater
(B) basket cells & stellate cells are seen
(C) axons and dendrites of stellate cells are confined to molecular layer
(D) all of the above

18. True about climbing fibers-
(A) are axons of inferior olivary nucleus
(B) synapse dendrites of purkinje cells
(C) terminal part of climbing fibers are seen in molecular layer
(D) all of the above

19. True about purkinje cell layer is-
(A) flask shaped cell body
(B) single layer of cells
(C) purkinje cell axons are only efferent fibers of cerebellum
(D) all of the above

20. True combination is-
(A) climbing fibers-efferent
(B) mossy fibers- efferent
(C) climbing fibers-afferent
(D) none of the above

21. Climbing fibers-
(A) originate from inferior olivary nucleus
(B) form excitatory synaptic contact with purkinje cells
(C) convey visual, somatosensory and cerebral cortical information
(D) all are true

22. Mossy fibers originate from-
(A) vestibular nuclei
(B) pontine nuclei
(C) spinal cord
(D) all of the above

23. True about cells in cerebellum is-
(A) purkinje cells-excitatory
(B) granule cells - excitatory
(C) basket cells - excitatory
(D) golgi cells -excitatory

24. True about cells in cerebellum is all except-
(A) purkinje cells-inhibitory
(B) basket cells - excitatory
(C) basket cells - inhibitory
(D) golgi cells -inhibitory

25. True about purkinje fibers is all except-
(A) efferent from cerebellar cotex
(B) generally terminate on cerebellar nuclie
(C) axons of purkinje cells are excitatory to cerebellar nuclei
(D) axons of purkinje cells are inhibitory to cerebellar nuclei

26. Cerebellar nuclei located anatomically medial to lateral-
(A) dentae-embliform-fastigial-globose
(B) embliform-fastigial-globose-dentae
(C) fastigial-globose-emboliform-dentate
(D) dentae-fastigial-globose-emboliform

27. True about fastigial nucleus is-
(A) part of archicerebellum
(B) vestibular in connection
(C) controls axial muscles in response to labyrinthine stimuli
(D) all of the above

28. True about dentate nucleus is all except-
(A) largest of cerebellar nuclei
(B) placed most medially among cerebellar nuclei
(C) hilum is directed anteromedially
(D) neocerebellar in connection

29. Wrong combination is-
(A) dentate nucleus-neocerebellum
(B) fastigial nucleus- archicerebellum
(C) globose & emboliformis – spinocerebellum
(D) fastigial nucleus-spinocerebellum

30. True about connections of dentate nucleus is all except-
(A) red nucleus
(B) thalamus
(C) hypothalamus
(D) inferior olivary nucleus

31. True about connections of emboliformis nucleus is all except-
(A) red nucleus
(B) thalamus
(C) inferior olivary nucleus
(D) pontine nuclei

32. True about connections of globose nucleus is all except-
(A) red nucleus
(B) superior colliculus
(C) hypothalamus
(D) thalamus

33. Arbor vitae is –
(A) seen in grey matter of cerebellum
(B) seen in white matter of cerebellum
(C) both of the above
(D) none of the above

34. Spinocerebellar syndrome may be due to-
(A) lesion of vermis
(B) medulloblastoma
(C) chronic alcoholism
(D) all of the above

35. Three cardinal signs of spinocerebellar syndrome are-
(A) ataxia-waddling gait
(B) cerebellar nystagmus
(C) speech disorders
(D) all of the above

36. Three cardinal signs of neocerebellar syndrome are-
(A) dysmetria
(B) intentional tremors
(C) hypotonia
(D) all of the above

37. Largest lobe of cerebellum is-
(A) anterior
(B) posterior
(C) flocculonodular lobe
(D) vermis

38. True about cerebellar peduncle is all except-
(A) superior cerebellar peduncle connects cerebellum to midbrain
(B) inferior cerebellar peduncle connects cerebellum to medulla
(C) middle cerebellar peduncle connects cerebellum to midbrain
(D) middle cerebellar peduncle connects cerebellum to pons

39. Most of the arterial supply to cerebellum comes from-
(A) basilar artery
(B) vertebral artery
(C) both
(D) none

40. Cerebellum is supplied by-
(A) anterior inferior cerebellar artery
(B) posterior inferior cerebellar artery
(C) superior cerebellar artery
(D) all of the above

Answer Sheet

1. C, 2. B, 3. A, 4. A, 5. C, 6. D, 7. D, 8. D, 9. B, 10. C, 11. A, 12. A, 13. A, 14. A, 15. D, 16. C, 17. D, 18. D, 19. D, 20. C, 21. D, 22. D, 23. B, 24. B, 25. C, 26. C, 27. D, 28. B, 29. D, 30. C, 31. C, 32. C, 33. B, 34. D, 35. D, 36. D, 37. B, 38. C, 39. C, 40. D

Chapter 8

Cerebrum

1. Cerebraum occupies –
   (A) anterior & middle cranial fossa
   (B) anterior & posterior cranial fossa
   (C) anterior, middle & posterior cranial fossa
   (D) middle & posterior cranial fossa
2. Surface area of cerebral surface is-
   (A) 1500-1750 cm^2
   (B) 1750-2000 cm^2
   (C) 2250-2500 cm^2
   (D) 3000 cm^2
3. Cavity of cerebrum is –
   (A) third ventricle
   (B) fourth ventricle
   (C) lateral ventricle
   (D) central canal
4. Inferior surface of cerebrum is divided into orbital & tentorial surface by-
   (A) central sulcus
   (B) stem of lateral sulcus
   (C) pre-occipital notch
   (D) pareito-occipital sulcus
5. Central sulcus begins-
   (A) just anterior to mid-point of supero-medial border
   (B) just posterior to mid-point of supero-medial border
   (C) at the mid-point of supero-medial border
   (D) none of the above
6. Fifth lobe of cerebral hemisphere is-
   (A) frontal lobe
   (B) insula
   (C) parietal lobe
   (D) hippocampal lobe
7. True about insula is-
   (A) consists of long and short gyri
   (B) separated by central sulcus of insula
   (C) lentiform nucleus lies deep to insular cortex
   (D) all of the above
8. Most medial gyrus on inferior surface is-
   (A) parahippocampal gyrus
   (B) medial occipito-temporal gyrus
   (C) Lateral occipito-temporal gyrus
   (D) uncus

9. Lingual gyrus is posterior continuation of-
(A) parahippocampal gyrus
(B) medial occipito-temporal gyrus
(C) Lateral occipito-temporal gyrus
(D) uncus

10. Sulci present on medial surface are all except-
(A) cingulate
(B) callosal
(C) interparietal
(D) calcarine

11. Sulci present on inferior surface are -
(A) orbital
(B) occipito-temporal
(C) olfactory
(D) all of the above

12. Cerebral cortex forms –
(A) 30% of mass of brain
(B) 40% of mass of brain
(C) 50% of mass of brain
(D) 60% of mass of brain

13. Cells seen in cerebral cortex are –
(A) pyramidal cells
(B) granule cells
(C) cells of martinotti
(D) all of the above

14. Cells seen in cerebral cortex are-
(A) fusiform cells
(B) basket cells
(C) horizontal cells of cajal
(D) all of the above

15. True about pyramidal cells is-
(A) form 2/3rd of cells in cerebral cortex
(B) tall & pyramidal in shape, apex pointing towards surface
(C) size 10 to 50 microns
(D) all are true

16. Betz cells are large pyramidal cells size 120 microns-seen in
(A) sensory cortex of cerebellum
(B) motor cortex of cerebrum
(C) sensory cortex of cerebrum
(D) motor cerebellar cortex

17. Axons of pyramidal cells form-
(A) association fibers
(B) commissural fibers
(C) projection fibers
(D) all of the above

18. Archicortex of cerebrum is seen in-
(A) frontal lobe
(B) hippocampal formation
(C) olfactory lobe
(D) limbic lobe

19. Paleocrtex of cerebrum –
(A) olfactory lobe
(B) limbic lobe (piriform lobe)
(C) consists of three to five layers
(D) all of the above

20. Brodmann divided cerebral cortex in-
(A) 43 areas
(B) 45 areas
(C) 47 areas
(D) 52 areas

21. Neocrtex of cerebrum consists of-
(A) six layers
(B) five to three layers
(C) three layers
(D) none of the above

22. Horizontal cells of Cajal are seen in-
(A) molecular layer
(B) external granular layer
(C) internal granular layer
(D) all of the above

23. External granular layer consists of-
(A) granular /stellate cells
(B) small pyramidal cells
(C) both
(D) none

24. External pyramidal layer consists of-
(A) pyramidal cells
(B) granular/stellate cells
(C) cells of martinotti
(D) all of the above

25. True about internal granular layer is-
(A) densly packed granule cells
(B) called outer layer of Baillarger
(C) seen in primary sensory cortex
(D) all are true

26. True about internal ganglionic (pyramidal) layer is-
(A) consists of betz and cells of Martinotti
(B) called internal layer of Baillarger
(C) seen in motor cortex
(D) all are true

27. All are true about granular cortex except -
(A) second & fourth layers are well developed
(B) sensory cortex
(C) motor cortex
(D) afferents from thalamus

28. All are true about Agranular cortex except -
(A) fifth layer is well developed
(B) motor cortex
(C) sensory cortex
(D) pyramidal cell layer is well developed

29. True about primary sensory area is all except-
(A) perceives pain, touch & temperature
(B) located in pre central gyrus area 3, 1, 2
(C) located in post central gyrus area 3, 1, 2
(D) gets afferent from thalamus

30. True about somatic sensory association area is all except-
(A) superior parietal lobule on lateral surface
(B) precuneus on medial surface
(C) lesion leads to stereognosis
(D) Brodmann's area 5 & 7

31. Brodmann's Area for taste sensation is-
(A) area 44
(B) area 45
(C) area 43
(D) area 47

32. Area for taste is located in-
(A) superior end of post central gyrus
(B) inferior end of post central gyrus
(C) posterior part of superior temporal gyrus
(D) none of the above

33. Vestibular area is located in-
(A) anterior end of intraparietal sulcus
(B) in the post central gyrus
(C) both
(D) none

34. True about sensory speech area of Wernike's is all except -
(A) located in dominant cerebral hemisphere
(B) located in posterior part of superior temporal gyrus

(C) area 22 & also functions as auditory association area
(D) located in posterior part of middle & inferior temporal gyrus

35. Broca's area is-
(A) area 44
(B) motor speech area
(C) connected with Wernike's area by arcuate fasciculus
(D) all of the above

36. Damage to parietal lobe may cause-
(A) aphasia
(B) apraxia
(C) ataxia
(D) astereognosis

37. Primary visual area is-
(A) area 17 of Brodmann's
(B) located on either side of calcarine sulcus
(C) medial aspect of occipital lobe on lingual gyrus & cuneus
(D) all of the above

38. True about line of Gennari is all except-
(A) inner band of Baillarger
(B) gives striated appearance to visual cortex
(C) on either side of calcarine sulcus
(D) outer band of Baillarger

39. True about visual association area is all except-
(A) area 18 & 19
(B) connects with frontal eye field & pulvinar
(C) causes conjugate eye movements to same side
(D) damage leads to visual agnosia

40. Heschl's gyrus is associated with-
(A) taste area
(B) primary auditory area
(C) sensory speech area
(D) all of the above

41. All are true about primary auditory area except –
(A) lies in the floor of lateral sulcus
(B) area 41 & 42
(C) receives afferent from medial geniculate body
(D) receives afferent from lateral geniculate body

42. Areas concerned with olfaction are –
(A) limen insuale
(B) uncus & entorhinal cortex
(C) amygdaloid body
(D) all of the above

43. True about primary motor area is-
(A) located in precentral gyrus & paracentral lobule
(B) area 4 of Broca
(C) predominance of pyramidal cells and scanty granular cells
(D) all of the above

44. Primary motor area contributes to pyramidal fibers-
(A) 30%
(B) 40%
(C) 50%
(D) 70%

45. Micturition centre is located in-
(A) parietal lobule
(B) paracentral lobule
(C) precuneus
(D) cuneus

46. Defaecation centre is located in-
(A) parietal lobule
(B) paracentral lobule
(C) precuneus
(D) cuneus

47. Supplementary motor area is-
(A) medial surface of cerebral cortex
(B) cingulate motor area is located adjacent to cingulate sulcus
(C) area 6
(D) all of the above

48. Damage to supplementary motor area leads to-
(A) spastic paralysis
(B) does not causes permanent loss
(C) both of above
(D) none of the above

49. True about premotor area is all except-
(A) posterior part of superior frontal gyrus
(B) posterior part of middle frontal gyrus
(C) posterior part of inferior frontal gyrus
(D) all of the above

50. Afferent to premotor area are from-
(A) sensory areas of cerebral cortex
(B) thalamus
(C) basal ganglion
(D) all of the above

51. All are true about premotor area except-
(A) directs the primary motor area to execute skilled movements
(B) controls postural movements through basal ganglion
(C) cortical centre for pyramidal system
(D) corresponds to area 6 of Brodmann

52. All are true about frontal eye field except-
(A) located in posterior part of superior frontal gyrus
(B) controls conjugate scanning movements of both eyes
(C) Brodmann's area 8
(D) located in posterior part of middle frontal gyrus

53. True about prefrontal cortex is all except-
(A) store house of all past experience
(B) controls behavior based on judgement & foresight
(C) controls motor movements of eye ball
(D) Brodmann's area 9,10,11,&12

54. True about motor speech area is all except-
(A) located in pars triangularis & pars opercularis in inferior frontal gyrus
(B) Brodmann's area 44 & 45
(C) located in dominant hemisphere
(D) located in pars triangularis & pars opercularis in superior temporal gyrus

55. Left cerebral hemisphere is responsible for all except -
(A) imagination and insight
(B) analytical skills
(C) mathematical calculations
(D) speech

56. Right cerebral hemisphere is responsible for all except -
(A) mathematical calculations
(B) imagination and insight
(C) musical awareness
(D) spatial perception

57. Visual association area is-
(A) area 17
(B) area 18
(C) area 19
(D) area 18 & 19

58. **Part of cerebral area recognizing toothache is-**
(A) precentral gyrus
(B) precuneus
(C) postcentral gyrus
(D) parietal lobule

59. **Motor speech area is located in-**
(A) superior temporal gyrus
(B) middle frontal gyrus
(C) inferior frontal gyrus
(D) none of the above

60. **Lesions of uncus are associated with-**
(A) visual hallucinations
(B) auditory hallucinations
(C) olfactory hallucinations
(D) none of the above

Answer Sheet

1. A, 2. C, 3. C, 4. B, 5. B, 6. B, 7. D, 8. A, 9. A, 10. C, 11. D, 12. B, 13. D, 14. D, 15. D, 16. B, 17. D, 18. B, 19. D, 20. D, 21. A, 22. A, 23. C, 24. D, 25. D, 26. D, 27. C, 28. C, 29. B, 30. C, 31. C, 32. B, 33. C, 34. D, 35. D, 36. B, 37. D, 38. A, 39. C, 40. B, 41. D, 42. D, 43. D, 44. A, 45. B, 46. B, 47. D, 48. C, 49. D, 50. D, 51. C, 52. A, 53. C, 54. D, 55. A, 56. A, 57. D, 58. C, 59. C, 60. C

Chapter 9

Ventricles & CSF

1. The 3rd ventricle is the cavity of the:
   (A) Metencephalon.
   (B) Mesencephalon.
   (C) Telencephalon.
   (D) Diencephalon.

2. The lateral ventricle communicates with the 3rd ventricle through:
   (A) Aqueduct of Sylvius.
   (B) Foramen of Magendie.
   (C) Foramen of Monro.
   (D) Foramen of Luschka.

3. The subarachnoid space:
   (A) Contains the cerebrospinal fluid.
   (B) Dilates in some areas to form the subarachnoid cisterns.
   (C) Subarachnoid hemorrhage is usually due to rupture of superficial cerebral veins.
   (D) All of the above are correct.

4. The lateral ventricle is the cavity of the:
   (A) Telencephalon.
   (B) Diencephalon.
   (C) Mesencephalon.
   (D) Rhombencephalon.

5. The central canal of the spinal cord opens out into the:
   (A) Subarachnoid space.
   (B) Sacral hiatus.
   (C) Third ventricle.
   (D) Fourth ventricle.

6. One of the following arteries is a branch of the basilar artery:
   (A) Anterior inferior cerebellar artery.
   (B) Posterior inferior cerebellar artery.
   (C) Anterior spinal artery.
   (D) Radicular arteries to the cervical part of the spinal cord.

7. The floor of the 4th ventricle is formed by the:
   (A) Superior medullary velum.
   (B) Inferior medullary velum.
   (C) Cerebellum.
   (D) Back of the medulla.

8. Regarding the CSF, one of the following is INCORRECT:
   (A) The main volume is present in the ventricles of the brain.
   (B) The choroid plexus is the main site of production.
   (C) The arachnoid villi and granulations are the main site of absorption (drainage).

(D) It reaches the subarachnoid space through the 3 foramina of the fourth ventricle.

9. The epithalamus is formed of all of the following EXCEPT:
(A) Habenular nucleus.
(B) Anterior commissure.
(C) Posterior commisure.
(D) Stria medullaris thalami.

10. The midbrain contains all of the following EXCEPT:
(A) Substantia nigra.
(B) Third ventricle.
(C) Oculomotor nerve nuclei.
(D) Trochlear nerve nucleus.

11. The epithalamus:
(A) Is part of the diencephalon.
(B) Contains a gland that secretes melatonin.
(C) Contains a nucleus that is part of the limbic system.
(D) All of the above are correct.

12. All of the following are correct EXCEPT:
(A) Area postrema is the vomiting center.
(B) The tuber cinereum of the interpeduncular fossa is part of the hypothalamus.
(C) The stria medullaris of the 4th ventricle are arcuatocerebellar fibers.
(D) Foramen of Megendie of the 4th ventricle is present in the superior medullary velum.

13. In the midbrain:
(A) The two superior colliculi are connected by the anterior commissure.
(B) The inferior brachium connects the inferior colliculus with the lateral geniculate body.
(C) The substantia nigra contains nerve cells that secrete noradrenaline.
(D) The posterior part (tectum) contains visual and auditory reflex centers.

14. Regarding the ventricular system, one of the following is INCORRECT:
(A) The ependymal lining contributes to the formation and circulation of the CSF.
(B) It contains about 30 ml of CSF.
(C) Obstruction of the aqueduct of Sylvius causes dilatation of all the ventricles.
(D) Communicates with subarachnoid space through foramina of Luschka and Megendie.

15. Nuclei of the limbic system include all of the following EXCEPT:
(A) Hippocampus.
(B) Amygdaloid nucleus.
(C) Caudate nucleus.
(D) Anterior thalamic nucleus

16. Language areas are located in all of the following EXCEPT:
(A) Supramarginal gyrus.
(B) Superior temporal gyrus.
(C) Middle frontal gyrus.
(D) Inferior frontal gyrus.

17. Regarding the anterior limb of the internal capsule, all the statements are correct EXCEPT:
(A) Contains the anterior thalamic radiation.
(B) Contains fibers from the anterior thalamic nucleus to the cingulate gyrus.
(C) Contains nonfrontopontine fibers.
(D) Supplied by branches of the anterior cerebral and middle cerebral arteries.

18. Regarding the ventricular system, one of the following is INCORRECT:

(A) it contains choroids plexus that secrete the CSF.

(B) it represents the cavity of the neural tube.

(C) it contains about 100 ml of CSF.

(D) obstruction of the aqueduct of Sylvius causes dilatation of the lateral and third ventricles.

19. Regarding the thalamic radiations, all are correct EXCEPT:

(A) the anterior thalamic radiation connects nuclei of the limbic system with the cerebral cortex.

(B) the inferior thalamic radiation carries auditory fibers to area 41 and 42.

(C) lesion in the posterior thalamic radiation causes contralateral homonymous hemianopia.

(D) lesion in the inferior thalamic radiation causes contralateral loss of hearing.

20. Regarding the thalamic nuclei, all are correct EXCEPT:

(A) The anterior nucleus is part of the limbic system.

(B) The medial nucleus is connected with the prefrontal cortex (personality center).

(C) The ventral anterior nucleus is connected with the motor and premotor areas.

(D) The ventral posterior lateral nucleus receives the medial lemniscus.

21. Regarding the medial geniculate body, all are correct EXCEPT:

(A) It receives auditory information from both ears but mainly from the opposite ear.

(B) It receives auditory information from the superior colliculus.

(C) It projects to the auditory area in the superior temporal gyrus.

(D) It projects through the sublenticular part of the internal capsule.

22. The hypothalamus:

(A) forms part of the mid-brain

(B) forms part of the roof of the third ventricle

(C) contains the tuber cinerueum

(D) has nerve connections with the anterior lobe of the pituitary gland

23. Which is ot true with regard to the internal capsule:

(A) it is made up of grey matter

(B) the anterior limb separates the caudate nucleus from the lenticular nucleus

(C) fibres connecting the frontal lobe to the red nucleus are found in the posterior limb

(D) contralateral spastic hemiplegia can result from infarction of the lenticulostriate artery

24. Which is not part of Pars dorsalis-

(A) Thalamus

(B) Epithalamus

(C) Metathalamus

(D) Subthalams

25. Which is subdivision of metathalamus

(A) Lateral geniculate body

(B) Habenular nuclei

(C) Subthalamic nucleus

(D) None of the above

26. Which is not true about pulvinar-

(A) It is anterior end of thalamus

(B) It overhangs geniculate bodies

(C) Related with superior colliculi

(D) None of the above

27. Which nuclei is not present in ventral tier group of laterapart of thalamus-
(A) Ventral anterior
(B) Ventral lateral
(C) Ventral medial
(D) Ventral anteromedial

28. The thalamic nucleus that receives pain and temperature sensations from the body is:
(A) The ventral posteromedial.
(B) The ventral posterolateral.
(C) The ventral anterior.
(D) The lateral geniculate.

29. The hypothalamic nucleus that controls the diurnal rhythm is:
(A) Paraventricular.
(B) Suprachiasmatic.
(C) Mammillary.
(D) Ventromedial.

30. Lateral geniculate body is –
(A) Anterolateral to medial geniculate body
(B) Larger than medial geniculate body
(C) Connected to inferior colliculus by superior brachium
(D) Grey matter consist of 5 layers.

31. Not true about pineal gland-
(A) Has no neural tissue.
(B) Supplied by nervus conarii
(C) Lesion of gland are associated with precocious puberty
(D) None of the above

32. True about boundaries of hypothalamus is –
(A) Posteriorly – subthalamus
(B) Medially – internal capsule
(C) Laterally – thalamus
(D) Superiorly – cavity of third ventricle

33. Which is not nucleus present in tuberal region of hypothalamus-
(A) Ventromedial nucleus
(B) Arcuate nucleus
(C) Dorsomedial nuclei
(D) Posterior nucleus

34. Third ventricle floor is formed by-
(A) Pineal gland
(B) Posterior commissure
(C) Lamina terminalis
(D) Mammillary body

35. Which recess of third ventricle is triangular-
(A) Optic recess
(B) Anterior recess
(C) Pineal recess
(D) Suprapineal recess

36. Which statement is not true-
(A) the foramen of Magendie is in the middle of the fourth ventricle
(B) the interpeduncular cistern lies behind the dorsum sella
(C) the third ventricle does not contain choroid plexus
(D) the pineal recess lies in the posterior aspect of the third ventricle

37. Motor fibres in Anterior limb of internal capsule are-
(A) Cortico nuclear
(B) Frontopontine
(C) Parietopontine
(D) Corticorubral

38. Charcot's artery of cerebral hemorrhage supplies-
(A) Anterior limb
(B) Posterior limb
(C) Genu
(D) Sub-lentiform part

39. Anterior choroidal artery is branch of-
(A) Posterior cerebral artery
(B) Internal carotid artery
(C) Anterior communicating artery
(D) Posterior communicating artery

40. Inferior thalamic radiation are also k/a-
(A) Auditory radiation
(B) Optic radiation
(C) Parietopontine fibres
(D) None of the above

Answer Sheet

1. D, 2. C, 3. D, 4. A, 5. D, 6. A, 7. D, 8. A, 9. B, 10. B, 11. D, 12. D, 13. A, 14. C, 15. C, 16. C, 17. C, 18. C, 19. D, 20. C, 21. B, 22. C, 23. A, 24. D, 25. A, 26. A, 27. D, 28. B, 29. B, 30. A, 31. D, 32. A, 33. D, 34. D, 35. B, 36. C, 37. B, 38. D, 39. B, 40. A

Chapter 10 Revision Test

Head, Neck & Brain

1. Correct about occipitofrontalis muscle is-
   (A) supplied by facial nerve
   (B) supplied by mandibular nerve
   (C) supplied by ophthalmic division of trigeminal nerve
   (D) all of the above

2. Surgical scalp is made up of-
   (A) skin & connective tissue
   (B) skin, connective tissue & epicranial aponeurosis
   (C) skin, connective tissue, epicranial aponeurosis & loose areolar tissue
   (D) skin, connective tissue, epicranial aponeurosis & pericranium

3. True about carotid canal is-
   (A) located on inferior surface of petrous temporal bone
   (B) internal carotid artery with sympathetic plexus around it
   (C) emissary vein connecting pharyngeal venous plexus to cavernous venous sinus
   (D) all of the above

4. Structure passing through tympanic canaliculus in jugular foramen is-
   (A) chorda tympani nerve
   (B) auricular branch of vagus nerve
   (C) tympanic branch of glossopharyngeal nerve
   (D) all of the above

5. Structures passing through foramen ovale are all except-
   (A) mandibular nerve
   (B) accessory middle meningeal artery
   (C) middle meningeal artery
   (D) lessor petrosal nerve

6. Structures passing through jugular foramen-
   (A) anterior part-inferior petrosal sinus
   (B) posterior part-sigmoid sinus
   (C) middle part-9th, 10th & 11th cranial nerves
   (D) all are true.

7. Structures passing through anterior condylar canal-
   (A) hypoglossal nerve
   (B) 12th cranial nerve & meningeal br of ascending pharyngeal artery
   (C) 11th & 12th cranial nerves
   (D) all of the above

8. Posterior part of foramen magnum gives way to all except-
(A) medulla oblongata with spinal root of accessory nerves
(B) 1 anterior & 2 posterior spinal arteries
(C) 2 vertebral arteries
(D) basilar artery

9. Distribution of phrenic nerve is-
(A) diaphragm
(B) diaphragmatic pleura
(C) pericardium
(D) all of the above

10. Largest branch of 1st part of subclavian artery is-
(A) inferior thyroid artery
(B) vertebral artery
(C) thyrocervical trunk
(D) internal thoracic artery

11. All are branches from thyro cervical trunk except-
(A) inferior thyroid artery
(B) suprascapular artery
(C) transverse scapular artery
(D) deep cervical artery

12. Vertebral artery passes through foramen transversarium of-
(A) C7 – C1
(B) C6 -- C1
(C) C7 – C2
(D) T1 – C1

13. Shortest branch of subclavian artery is-
(A) inferior thyroid artery
(B) vertebral artery
(C) thyrocervical trunk
(D) internal thoracic artery

14. Occasionally clavicle is pierced by –
(A) medial supraclavicular nerve
(B) middle supraclavicular nerve
(C) lateral supraclavicular nerve
(D) all of the above

15. During lymph node removal /biopsy in posterior triangle of neck nerve most commonly damaged is-
(A) lesser occipital nerve
(B) great auricular nerve
(C) spinal accessory nerve
(D) supraclavicular nerve

16. Virchow's lymph nodes are-
(A) right supraclavicular lymph nodes
(B) left supraclavicular lymph nodes
(C) right subclavicular lymph nodes
(D) left subclavicular lymph nodes

17. Commonest cause of cervical lymphadenopathy in adults-
(A) cancer
(B) scalp infection
(C) cervical abscess
(D) meningitis

18. Sternocleidomastoid is supplied by-
(A) spinal accessory nerve
(B) C2 & C3 nerve
(C) Both
(D) cranial accessory nerve

19. Articular disc of TMJ is made up of-
(A) Fibrocartilage
(B) Fibrous tissue
(C) Hyaline cartilage
(D) Articular cartilage

20. Wrong srtatement is-
(A) subclavian vein passes posterior to sclaneus anterior
(B) subclavian artery passes posterior to sclaneus anterior

(C) lower trunk of brachial plexus passes posterior to sclaneus anterior
(D) subclavian vein passes anterior to sclaneus anterior

21. Posterior most part-Root- of the tongue – sensory supply is-
(A) lingual nerve
(B) glosso pharyngeal nerve
(C) superior laryngeal nerve
(D) hypoglossal nerve

22. Anterior 2/3 of the tongue –sensory supply is-
(A) lingual nerve
(B) vagus nerve
(C) glossopharyngeal nerve
(D) hypoglossal nerve

23. Anterior 2/3 of the tongue is supplied by-
(A) lingual nerve + chorda tympani nerve
(B) chorda tympani nerve + glossopharyngeal nerve
(C) glossopharyngeal nerve + vagus nerve
(D) none of the above

24. Posterior 1/3 of the tongue is supplied by-
(A) lingual nerve + chorda tympani nerve
(B) chorda tympani nerve + glossopharyngeal nerve
(C) glossopharyngeal nerve + vagus nerve
(D) glossopharyngeal nerve + hypoglossal nerve

25. Taste sensations from anterior 2/3 of the tongue is carried by-
(A) lingual nerve
(B) chorda tympani nerve
(C) glossopharyngeal nerve
(D) B+C

26. Taste sensations from posterior 1/3 of the tongue is carried by-
(A) lingual nerve
(B) chorda tympani nerve
(C) glossopharyngeal nerve
(D) hypoglossal nerve

27. General & taste sensations from anterior 2/3 of tongue is carried by
(A) lingual nerve + chorda tympani nerve
(B) chorda tympani nerve + glossopharyngeal nerve
(C) lingual +chorda tympani nerve + glossopharyngeal nerve
(D) glossopharyngeal nerve + vagus + hypoglossal nerve

28. Parotid duct opens into vestibule of mouth-
(A) opposite to crown of 2nd mandibular premolar
(B) opposite to crown of 2nd mandibular molar
(C) opposite to crown of 2nd maxillary molar
(D) opposite to crown of 2nd maxillary premolar

29. Structures pierced by parotid duct are all except-
(A) buccal pad of fat & buccopharyngeal fascia
(B) buccinators muscle
(C) pharyngobasilar fascia
(D) buccal mucosa

30. Ducts of sublingual glands are called -
(A) Wharton's duct
(B) Stensen's duct
(C) duct of Rivinus
(D) none

31. Submandibular gland develops from-
(A) ectooderm
(B) mesoderm
(C) endoderm
(D) all

32. Arterial wall of middle ear cavity is-
(A) anterior wall
(B) posterior wall
(C) floor
(D) posterior wall

33. Secretomotor fibers to lacrimal gland are through-
(A) pterygopalatine ganglion
(B) parotid ganglion
(C) submandibular ganglion
(D) ciliary ganglion

34. Secretomotor nerve for parotid gland is–
(A) facial nerve
(B) glossopharyngeal nerve
(C) vagus nerve
(D) none of the above

35. Parotid gland start developing at-
(A) 6th week of intrauterine life
(B) 7th week of intrauterine life
(C) 8th week of intrauterine life
(D) 9th week of intrauterine life

36. Lymphatics draining tongue are mainly -
(A) sub mandibular lymph nodes
(B) sub mental lymph nodes
(C) juglodigastric lymph nodes
(D) juglo omohyoid lymph nodes

37. All are true about capsules of thyroid gland except-
(A) true capsule is formed by condensation of fibrous stroma of gland
(B) false capsule is made up of pretracheal layer of deep fascia
(C) venous plexus lies between true & false capsule
(D) venous plexus lies beneath the true capsule

38. Artery of first branchial arch is-
(A) mandibular nerve
(B)-mandibular artery
(C)-maxillary artery
(D)-Stapedial artery

39. All are true about venous drainage of thyroid gland is except -
(A) superior thyroid veins drain into IJV of respective side
(B) middle thyroid veins drain into IJV of respective side
(C) fourth thyroid veins or vein of Kocher Drains into IJV of respective side
(D) inferior thyroid veins drain into brachiocephalic veins of respective side

40. Epithelium of thyroid gland is-
(A) cuboidal
(B) simple squamous
(C) columnar
(D) all of the above

41. All are true about mandible except-
(A) angle is 110^0 in adults
(B) angle is 160^0 in children
(C) angle is 140^0 in old age
(D) membranocartilagenous in ossification

42. TMJ is supplied by-
(A) auriculotemporal n
(B) massetric n
(C) both A & B
(D) Auriculotemporal n, massetric n & C1 from cervical plexus

43. Buccinators is supplied by-
(A) mandibular n
(B) facial n
(C) glossopharyngeal n
(D) nerve to mylohyoid

44. Retraction of mandible is done by-
(A) masseter
(B) lateral pterygoid
(C) temporalis
(D) medial pterygoid

45. Action of the lateral pterygoid muscle is-
(A) closing of mouth
(B) opening of mouth
(C) retraction of lower jaw
(D) clenching of the teeth

46. All ligaments are derivatives of branchial arches except-
(A) stylohyoid ligament
(B) sphenomandibular ligament
(C) stylomandibular ligament
(D) anterior ligament of malleus

47. Sphenomandibular ligament is pierced by -
(A) mental nerve
(B) massetric nerve
(C) mylohyoid nerve
(D) none of the above

48. Most common nerve block in dental practice-
(A) lingual nerve
(B) inferior alveolar nerve
(C) mandibular nerve
(D) mylohyoid nerve

49. Most common direction of TMJ dislocation is-
(A) posterior
(B) anterior
(C) inferior
(D) postero-inferior

50. Muscle of head and neck called as Peripheral heart is-
(A) medial pterygoid
(B) lateral pterygoid
(C) medial & lateral pterygoid both
(D) temporalis

51. Protraction & Retraction of jaw at TMJ is done in –
(A) lower compartment
(B) upper compartment
(C) both compartments
(D) none of the above

52. Largest division of trigeminal nerve is-
(A) mandibular division
(B) maxillary division
(C) ophthalmic division
(D) auriculo-temporal nerve

53. Opening in superior meatus is-
(A) nasolacrimal duct
(B) anterior ethmoidal sinus
(C) posterior ethmoidal sinus
(D) middle ethmoidal sinus

54. Structures opening in middle meatus are-
(A) maxillary sinus
(B) frontal sinus
(C) middle & anterior ethmoidal sinuses
(D) all of the above

55. Sinus opening on bulla ethmoidalis-
(A) maxillary sinus
(B) frontal sinus
(C) anterior ethmoidal sinuses
(D) middle ethmoidal sinus

56. Viens of the nasal cavity drain into-
(A) pterygoid venous plexus
(B) pharyngeal venous plexus
(C) facial vein
(D) all of the above

57. Skull is made up of-
(A) 22 bones
(B) 28 bones
(C) 14 bones
(D) 20 bones

58. All are paired cartilage of larynx except-
(A) arytenoid
(B) cricoid
(C) corniculate
(D) cuneiform

59. Chorda tympani nerve is-
(A) post trematic nerve of first branchial arch
(B) post trematic nerve of second branchial arch
(C) pre trematic nerve of first branchial arch
(D) all of the above

60. Structures passing through sinus of Morgagni-
(A) auditory tube
(B) levator palate muscle
(C) ascending palatine & palatine branch of ascending pharyngeal artery
(D) all of the above

61. Structures passing through between superior & middle constrictor
(A) auditory tube
(B) levator palati muscle
(C) glossopharyngeal nerve & levator palate
(D) glossopharyngeal nerve & stylopharyngeus

62. Structures passing between middle & inferior constrictor-
(A) internal laryngeal nerve & inferior laryngeal artery
(B) superior laryngeal nerve & superior laryngeal artery
(C) external laryngeal nerve & superior laryngeal artery
(D) internal laryngeal nerve & superior laryngeal artery

63. Structures passing through inferior constrictor & oesophagus -
(A) recurrent laryngeal nerve & inferior laryngeal artery
(B) recurrent laryngeal nerve & superior laryngeal artery
(C) internal laryngeal nerve & superior laryngeal artery
(D) recurrent laryngeal nerve & inferior laryngeal artery

64. Pharyngeal plexus is located on-
(A) superior constrictor muscle
(B) middle constrictor muscle
(C) inferior constrictor muscle
(D) all of the above

65. Neurons seen in dorsal nerve root ganglion are-
(A) bipolar
(B) pseudounipolar / unipolar
(C) multipolar
(D) anaxonic

66. Bipolar neurons are seen in-
(A) spiral ganglion of vestibular nerve
(B) retina
(C) olfactory neuroepithelium
(D) all of the above

67. Pseudo unipolar neurons are seen in-
(A) mesencephalic nucleus of trigeminal nerve
(B) dorsal root ganglia of spinal nerves
(C) sensory ganglion of cranial nerves
(D) all of the above

68. Diameter of spinal cord is minimum at–
(A) cervical region
(B) thoracic region
(C) lumbar region
(D) sacral region

69. Lower border of spinal cord terminates at-
(A) L1
(B) L2
(C) T12
(D) S1

70. Cervical enlargement extends –
(A) C3 to T1 spinal cord segment
(B) C4 to T1 spinal cord segment
(C) C4 to T2 spinal cord segment
(D) C5 to T1 spinal cord segment

71. Lumbar enlargement extends –
(A) L1 to S1 spinal cord segment
(B) L1 to S2 spinal cord segment
(C) L1 to S3 spinal cord segment
(D) L2 to S4 spinal cord segment

72. Conus medullaris lies at the-
(A) T12 Vertebral level
(B) L1 Vertebral level
(C) L2 Vertebral level
(D) L3 Vertebral level

73. True about antero-median fissure of spinal cord is-
(A) 3 mm deep
(B) lodges anterior spinal artery
(C) reaches up to grey commissure
(D) all of the above

74. True about nucleus proprious is-
(A) gives origin to ventral spinothalamic tract
(B) present in entire length
(C) corresponds to lamina 3 & 4
(D) all of the above

75. True about inferior colliculus is all except-
(A) large nucleus of auditory pathway
(B) afferent from lateral lemniscus
(C) efferents to lateral geniculate body
(D) efferents to medial geniculate body

76. All are true about Edinger Westphal nucleus except-
(A) visceral motor nucleus at inferior colliculus
(B) preganglionic parasympathetic fibers reach ciliary ganglion
(C) supplies ciliaris muscle
(D) supplies constrictor pupillae muscle of iris

77. All are true for Red Nucleus except –
(A) seen at upper level of midbrain
(B) contains copper rich pigment
(C) part of extrapyramidal system
(D) motor nucleus and controls posture & muscle tone

78. Lemniscus not seen at superior colliculus is-
(A) medial lemniscus
(B) lateral lemniscus
(C) trigeminal lemniscus
(D) spinal lemniscus

79. Weber's syndrome is due to occlusion of-
(A) anterior cerebral artery
(B) posterior cerebral artery
(C) middle cerebral artery
(D) posterior inferior cerebellar artery

80. Trochlear nerve-
(A) originates from the dorsal aspect of brain
(B) runs across lateral aspect of crus cerebri
(C) runs between superior cerebellar and posterior cerebral arteries
(D) all are true

81. Brachium of superior colliculus-
(A) bands of white fibers
(B) connects optic tract & lateral geniculate body
(C) conveys visual impulses
(D) all are true

82. Cranial nerve arising from medial side of crus cerebri is-
(A) optic nerve
(B) olfactory nerve
(C) oculomotor nerve
(D) trochlear nerve

83. Archicerebellum is-
(A) vestibular in connection
(B) flocculonodular lobe is main part
(C) responsible for maintenance of posture and balance
(D) all of the above

84. True about lateral zone is all except-
(A) controls muscle tone
(B) largest zone of cerebellum
(C) co-ordinates motor activities
(D) dentate in connection

85. True about cells in cerebellum is-
(A) purkinje cells-excitatory
(B) granule cells - excitatory
(C) basket cells - excitatory
(D) golgi cells –excitatory

86. Cerebellum is supplied by-
(A) anterior inferior cerebellar artery
(B) posterior inferior cerebellar artery
(C) superior cerebellar artery
(D) all of the above

87. Largest lobe of cerebellum is-
(A) anterior lobe
(B) posterior lobe
(C) flocculonodular lobe
(D) vermis

88. Brodmann divided cerebral cortex in-
(A) 43 areas
(B) 45 areas
(C) 47 areas
(D) 52 areas

89. Brodmann's Area for taste sensation is-
(A) area 44
(B) area 45
(C) area 43
(D) area 41

90. True about sensory speech area of Wernike's is all except -
(A) located in dominant cerebral hemisphere
(B) located in posterior part of superior temporal gyrus
(C) area 22 & also functions as auditory association area
(D) located in posterior part of middle & inferior temporal gyrus

91. Broca's area is-
(A) area 44 & 45
(B) motor speech area
(C) connected with Wernike's area by arcuate fasciculus
(D) all of the above

92. Damage to parietal lobe may cause-
(A) aphasia
(B) apraxia
(C) ataxia
(D) astereognosis

93. Area for smell is-
(A) 28
(B) 43
(C) 22
(D) 5 & 7

94. Tensor tympani muscle is supplied by-
(A) maxillary n
(B) mandibular n
(C) glossopharyngeal n
(D) facial n

95. Tympanic plexus is formed by-
(A) mandibular n
(B) facial n
(C) glossopharyngeal n
(D) vagus n

96. All pass through lateral wall of cavernous venous sinus except-
(A) occulomotor n
(B) trochlear n
(C) abduscent n
(D) ophthalmic division of trigeminal n

97. Pre trematic nerve of second arch is-
(A) mandibular n
(B) jacobson'n
(C) vagus n
(D) facial n

98. Vidian nerve is formed by-
(A) by joining greater superficial petrosal n & lesser petrosal n
(B) by joining deep petrosal n & greater superficial petrosal n
(C) by joining deep petrosal n & lesser superficial petrosal n
(D) all of the above

99. Regarding the medial geniculate body, all are correct EXCEPT:
(A) it receives auditory information from both ears but mainly from the opposite ear.
(B) it receives auditory information from the superior colliculus.
(C) it projects to the auditory area in the superior temporal gyrus.
(D) it projects through the sublenticular part of the internal capsule.

100. The thalamic nucleus that receives pain and temperature sensations from the head and neck is:
(A) the ventral posterolateral.
(B) the ventral posteromedial.
(C) the ventral anterior.
(D) the lateral geniculate

Answer Sheet

1. A (Occipito frontalis is muscle of facial expression & all muscles of facial expression are supplied by facial nerve), **2.** B (Upper three layers are a single unit and are avulsed together in injury or accidents sutured together as on unit called as surgical scalp), **3.** D, **4.** C (Tympanic branch of glossopharyngeal nerve passes through it and via floor of tympanic cavity reaches and joins tympanic plexus at promontory of medial wall of cavity), **5.** C (MALE-ie mandibular n, accessory meningeal artery, lessor petrosal nerve & emissiary vein passes through foramen ovale. middle meningeal artery passes through foramen spinosum), **6.** D, **7.** B (Anterior condylar canal is also known as hypoglossal canal), **8.** D (Two vertebral arteries enter foramen magnum and inside cranium unite in front of pons as basilar artery), **9.** D, **10.** B, **11.** D, **12.** B (Vertebral artery has four parts, 1st in sclaneo vertebral triangle, 2nd in foramen transversarium of C6 To C1, 3rd in Occipital triangle & 4th intracranial part. Remember that foramen transversarium of C7 gives passage to Vertebral Vein & Sympathetic plexus around it), **13.** C, **14.** B (Clavicle is also called as Dermal bone), **15.** C (Most superficial nerve here is spinal accessory & supplies sternocleido-mastoid & trapezius), **16.** B, **17.** A (Most common cancers are of oral cavity and upper respiratory tracts leading to metas-tasis and cervical lymphadenopathy), **18.** C, **19.** B (Articular disc is made up of FIBROUS TISSUE only after the age of 40 years it may convert to fibrocartilage), **20.** A (Subclavian vein is anterior to muscle while subclavian artery & lower trunk of brachial plexus are deep or posterior to it), **21.** C (Root or fixed posterior part of tongue is developed from fourth branchial arch and so supplied by superior laryngeal nerve – branch of vagus as nerve of fourth arch), **22.** A (Anterior 2/3 is developed from two lingual swellings derived from first branchial arch and so lingual branch of mandibular nerve – nerve of first arch supplies it), **23.** D (Anterior 2/3 motor-hypoglossal n, sensory-Lingual, taste-chorda tympani, taste – for- circumvallate papilla- Glossopharyngeal nerve & area of circumvallate papilla for general sensa-tion- glossopharyngeal nerve), **24.** D (Post part 1/3, develops from third arch and muscles come from occipital myotomes so supplied by 9th & 12th cranial nn), **25.** D, **26.** C, **27.** C, **28.** C (Upper 2nd molar is fixed bony point), **29.** C (Pharyngo basilar fascia is innermost covering of pharynx), **30.** C, **31.** C (Parotid is ectodermal while submandibular & sublingual glands are endodermal in origin), **32.** A (Anterior wall is only wall of middle ear cavity related to internal carotid artery), **33.** A, **34.** B, **35.** A, **36.** D (Main lymph nodes of tonsil are juglodigastric while main or principal lymph nodes for tongue are juglo omohyohyoid), **37.** C (Venous plexus in case of thyroid gland is deep to true capsule and is situated in between true & false capsule in case of prostate), **38.** C (Nerve of 1st branchial arch is mandibular nerve and artery of the arch is maxillary artery), **39.** D (Inferior thyroid veins of both side either right or left side drain into LEFT BRACHIOCEPHALIC VEIN because of horizontal course), **40.** D (Acco-rding to activity of gland epithelium chan-ges like in hyper active state- columnar, active state–cuboidal & inactive or resting phase–simple squamous), **41.** B (Angle is 110 in adults and 140 in both children and old age the difference is only location of mental foramen location near base in children and near alveolar margin in old age), **42.** C, **43.** B. (Buccinator is muscle of facial expression and so supplied by Buccal branch of facial nerve but skin and mucosa covering over it is supplied by Buccal branch of Mandibular nerve which is sensory), **44.** C, **45.** B, **46.** C (Spheno-mandibular ligament & anterior ligament of malleus – first arch, stylohyoid liga-ment- second arch, while stylomandibular ligament is condensation of investing layer of deep cervical fascia, seprates parotid gland and submandibular gland) **47.** C, **48.** B, **49.** B, **50.** B, **51.** B, **52.** A, **53.** C, **54.** D, **55.** D, **56.** D, **57.** B, **58.** B, **59.** C (Post trematic nerve for first arch is Mandibular nerve & pre trematic nerve is chorda tympani nerve), **60.** D, **61.** D, **62.** D, **63.** D, **64.** B, **65.** B, **66.** D (Peripheral process of bipolar neurons act like receptors and central processes form nerve), **67.** D, **68.** B (Max diametr is in cervical region and minimum in thoracic region), **69.** A, **70.** C, **71.** C, **72.** B, **73.** D, **74.** D, **75.** C (Inferior colliculus, medial geniculate body, lateral lemniscus and trapezoid body all are part of auditory pathway while superior colliculus & lateral geniculate body are part of visual pathway), **76.** A (Occulomotor nu, Edinger Westphal nu & red nucleus are seen at upper level or superior colliculus level of mid brain), **77.** B, **78.** B (Lateral lemniscus finishes and joins and terminates in inferior colliculus so not seen at superior colliculus), **79.** B, **80.** D, **81.** D (Superior colliculus & lateral geniculate body are in the pathway of vision), **82.** C (3rd cranial nerve arises from medial side of crus cerebri while 4th cranial nerve from lateral side of crus cerebri), **83.** D, **84.** A, **85.** B (All cerebellar cells are inhibitory except for granule cells which are excitatory). **86.** D, **87.** B, **88.** C, **89.** C, **90.** D, **91.** D, **92.** B, **93.** A, **94.** B, **95.** C, **96.** C, **97.** B (Tympanic branch of glossopharyngeal nerve is pre trematic nerve of second branchial arch), **98.** B, **99.** B, **100.** B (Pain and temperature reaches to VPL i.e. Ventro Postero Lateral nucleus but in case of Head Neck and Face it reaches in VPM ie Ventro Postero Medial nucleus of Thalamus).

Section - 3

Embryology

Chapter 1

Chromosomes and Cell Divisions

1. The stages of development are -
(A) embryonic and foetal
(B) germinal, embryonic and foetal
(C) germinal and foetal
(D) embryonic only

2. Embryo is the stage of development –
(A) first two months of intrauterine life
(B) third months onwards of intrauterine life
(C) nine months of intrauterine life
(D) first four months of intrauterine life

3. Germinal period is the stage of development –
(A) first three weeks of intrauterine life
(B) fourth week to eighth week onwards of intrauterine life
(C) first two months of intrauterine life
(D) first four months of intrauterine life

4. Foetal period is the stage of development –
(A) first two months of intrauterine life
(B) third months onwards of intrauterine life
(C) nine months of intrauterine life
(D) first four months of intrauterine life

5. What are the basic processes of development?
(A) growth and differentiation
(B) growth and determination
(C) growth, determination and differentiation
(D) growth, determination, migration and differentiation

6. The gonads produce -
(A) primordial sex cells only
(B) primordial sex cells and sex hormones
(C) sex hormones only
(D) develop primordial sex cells and also sex hormones

7. What describes number of chromosomes and amount of DNA in a gamete?
(A) 46 chromosomes (1n)
(B) 46 chromosomes (2n)
(C) 23 chromosomes (1n)
(D) 23 chromosomes (2n)

8. What is the main result of mitotic cell division?
(A) formation of two daughter cells with diploid (2n) number of chromosomes
(B) formation of two daughter cells with haploid (1n) number of chromosomes
(C) genetic exchange
(D) formation of duplicated chromosomes

9. In mitotic cell division, DNA replication of each chromosome occurs during interphase resulting in structure consisting of two chromatids. What is the structure known as -
(A) A duplicated chromosomes
(B) Two chromosomes
(C) A synapsed chromosomes
(D) A homologous pair

10. What is the main result of meiotic cells division?
(A) formation of two daughter cells with diploid number of chromosomes
(B) formation of daughter cells with haploid number of chromosomes with genetic variability
(C) genetic variability
(D) restoration of diploid number of chromosomes

11. A normal somatic cell contains -
(A) 22 autosomes and a sex chromosomes
(B) 23 autosomes and a sex chromosomes
(C) 22 autosomes
(D) 22 pair of autosomes and a pair of sex chromosomes

12. At which stage of meiotic cell division "crossing over" takes place -
(A) metaphase of 1st meiotic division
(B) laptotene of prophase of 1st meiotic division
(C) second meiotic division
(D) at time of formation of gamete

13. Foetal sex can be determined by noting presence or absence of Barr body in cells obtained from amniotic fluid. What is aetiology of Barr body -
(A) inactivation of both X chromosomes
(B) inactivation of homologous chromosomes
(C) inactivation of one X chromosomes
(D) inactivation of Y chromosomes

14. Gametes are derived from primordial germ cells from yolk sac at-
(A) 3rd week of intrauterine life
(B) 4th week of intrauterine life
(C) 6th week of intrauterine life
(D) 8th week of intrauterine life

15. Growth pattern seen in human embryo is-
(A) multiplicative
(B) auxetic
(C) accretic
(D) all of the above

16. Primary organiser region of embryo is-
(A) notochord
(B) primitive streak & node
(C) paraxial mesoderm
(D) none of the above

17. First and foremost differentiation during development is-
(A) chemo - differentiation
(B) histo - differentiation
(C) organo - differentiation
(D) none of the above

18. Features of prophase are-
(A) chromatids are thread like
(B) later acquire rod like shape
(C) in end stage chromosomes become quite distinct
(D) all of the above

19. Features of metaphase are-
(A) centrioles appear and move to opposite poles
(B) spindle formation
(C) disintegration of nuclear membrane
(D) all of the above

20. Features of metaphase are-
(A) chromosomes move to equator
(B) through centromere chromosomes get attached to spindle
(C) nucleoli disappears
(D) all of the above

21. Centrioles and spindle is typical of -
(A) anaphase
(B) prophase
(C) metaphase
(D) telophase

22. In anaphase number of chromosomes is-
(A) 46 chromosomes
(B) 46 pairs of chromosomes
(C) 23 chromosomes
(D) none of the above

23. Features of telophase are-
(A) two daughter nuclei
(B) centrioles are duplicated
(C) cells organelles are duplicated
(D) all of the above

24. Laptotene, zygotene, pachytene & diplotene are part of-
(A) prophase
(B) metaphase
(C) anaphase
(D) telophase

25. Bivalent or synopsis of chromosomes is seen in-
(A) leptotene
(B) zygotene
(C) pachytene
(D) diplotene

26. Tetrad or synopsis of chromosomes is seen in-
(A) leptotene
(B) zygotene
(C) pachytene
(D) diplotene

27. Crossing over of chromosomes is seen in-
(A) leptotene
(B) zygotene
(C) pachytene
(D) diplotene

28. Generally in utero life of any individual is-
(A) 266 days
(B) 240 days
(C) 275 days
(D) none of the above

29. DNA contains following bases-
(A) adenine, guanine & cytosine
(B) adenine, guanine, cytosine & uracil
(C) adenine, guanine, cytosine & thymine
(D) guanine, cytosine, uracil & thymine

30. RNA contains following bases-
(A) adenine, guanine & cytosine
(B) adenine, guanine, cytosine & uracil
(C) adenine, guanine, cytosine & thymine
(D) guanine, cytosine, uracil & thymine

31. Karyotyping is done on –
(A) lymphoid tissue sample
(B) bone marrow
(C) blood sample
(D) oral mucosa

32. Karyotyping is done on –
(A) lymphocytes
(B) red blood cells
(C) neutrophils
(D) fibroblasts/cytesm

Answer Sheet

1. (B)	2. (A)	3. (A)	4. (B)	5. (D)	6. (D)	7. (C)	8. (A)	9. (A)	10. (B)
11. (D)	12. (B)	13. (C)	14. (B)	15. (D)	16. (B)	17. (A)	18. (D)	19. (D)	20. (D)
21. (C)	22. (B)	23. (D)	24. (A)	25. (B)	26. (C)	27. (C)	28. (A)	29. (C)	30. (B)
31. (C)	32. (A)								

EXPLANATIONS

1. **(B)** The stage of development are germinal period-(from fertilisation up to 3rd week i.e formation of three primary germinal layer), embryonic period (from 4th to 8th week) and foetal period (from 3rd month up to birth of child)

5. **(D)** The basic processes of development are growth, determination i.e fixation of fates of different parts of embryo, migration i.e movement of cells to their prospective parts and differentiation i.e formation of new type of cells from existing ones.

6. **(D)** The gonads (sex glands) develop primordial sex cells (from walls of yolk sac). They also produce sex hormones that are responsible for development of reproductive organs and secondary sexual characters.

7. **(C)** The gametes or sex cells contain 23 chromosomes and n number of DNA. When two gametes fuse at fertilisation a zygote contains 46 chromosomes and 2n number of DNA.

8. **(A)** The main result of mitotic cells division is formation of two daughter cells with 2n number of chromosomes.

9. **(A)** During mitotic cell division, the DNA replication results in formation of two chromatids in each chromosome. The structure of chromosomes is then known as duplicated chromosomes.

10. **(B)** The main result of miotic cell division is formation of daughter cells with haploid (n) number of chromosomes and genetic variability that occurs during "crossing over"

11. **(D)** A normal somatic cell contains 22 pairs of autosomes and a pair of sex chromosomes that may be XX (in female) or XY (in male).

12. **(B)** The 'crossing over' or the exchange of genetic material in a segment of chromosomes takes place during Leptotene of prophase of 1st meiotic division.

13. **(C)** Foetal sex can be determined by noting the presence of "Barr body" in cells obtained from amniotic fluid. The Barr body is formed by inactivation of one X chromosomes.

Chapter 2

Male Sex Glands – Testes and Spermatogenesis

1. Where do the primordial sex cells develop-
   (A) In walls of yolk sac during 4th week of intra-uterine life
   (B) Inside gonads at birth
   (C) In walls of yolk sac during 5th week of intra-uterine life
   (D) Inside gonads at puberty
2. Approximately how many sperms are ejaculated by a normal fertile male during sexual intercourse-
   (A) 10 million
   (B) 20 million
   (C) 100 million
   (D) 350 million
3. In production of male gametes, which of the following cells remain dormant for 12-14 years-
   (A) Primordial germ cells
   (B) Primary spermatocyte
   (C) Secondary spermatocyte
   (D) Spermatid
4. When does formation of primary spermatocyte begin-
   (A) During 4th week of intra-uterine life
   (B) During 5th month of intra-uterine life
   (C) At birth
   (D) At puberty
5. How much DNA a primary spermatocyte contain-
   (A) 1n (B) 2n
   (C) 4n (D) 6n
6. The male hormone testosterone is secreted by-
   (A) Sertoli cells
   (B) Spermatogonia
   (C) Leydig cells
   (D) Epididymis
7. The head part of spermatozoon is formed by which part of spermatid-
   (A) Centriole
   (B) Mitochondria
   (C) Cytoplasm
   (D) Nucleus

8. Spermiogenesis is –
(A) formation of primary spermatocyte
(B) formation of secondary spermatocyte
(C) formation of spermatozoa from spermatids
(D) formation of spermatids

9. Spermatogenesis is –
(A) formation of primary spermatocyte
(B) formation of sperm from primordial germ cell
(C) formation of spermatozoa from spermatids
(D) formation of spermatids

10. Average number of spermatozoa in semen is-
(A) 20 million per ml
(B) 20 - 50 million per ml
(C) 50 – 150 million per ml
(D) 200 - 350 million per ml

11. Infertile male are having Sperm counts less than -
(A) 20 million per ml
(B) 20 - 50 million per ml
(C) 50 – 150 million per ml
(D) 200 - 350 million per ml

12. Function of Sertoli cells is-
(A) nourishment of sperms
(B) regulating the cell division in germ cells
(C) phagocytosis of residual bodies
(D) all of the above

13. In germinal epithelium spermatogonia are seen in-
(A) outermost layer
(B) intermediate layer
(C) inner most layer
(D) all of the above

14. In germinal epithelium spermatocytes are seen in-
(A) outermost layer
(B) intermediate layer
(C) inner most layer
(D) all of the above

15. In germinal epithelium spermatids are seen in-
(A) outermost layer
(B) intermediate layer
(C) inner most layer
(D) all of the above

16. Spermatogenesis takes place in –
(A) seminiferous tubules
(B) seminal vesicles
(C) vas differentia
(D) all of the above

17. Spermatogenesis takes place in seminiferous tubules of testis under the influence of-
(A) FSH
(B) testosterone
(C) estrogen
(D) progesterone

18. Spermatogenesis begins –
(A) before birth
(B) at puberty
(C) after puberty is over
(D) after the 21 years of age

19. Spermatogonia from birth till puberty remain in-
(A) resting phase
(B) proliferative phase
(C) A & B both
(D) none of the above

20. Spermatogonia at puberty remain in-
(A) resting phase
(B) proliferative phase
(C) A & B both
(D) none of the above

21. Seminiferous tubules are formed by canalization of sex cords of testis at the-
(A) from birth till prepuberty
(B) at puberty
(C) after puberty
(D) none of the above

22. Time taken in transformation of primary spermatogonia into primary spermatocyte is –
(A) 2 weeks
(B) 5 weeks
(C) 7 weeks
(D) 9 weeks

23. One B spermatogonia gives rise to –
(A) 4 spermatocytes
(B) 8 spermatocytes
(C) 16 spermatocytes
(D) 32 spermatocytes

24. Each primary spermatocyte gives rise to –
(A) 4 spermatids
(B) 8 spermatids
(C) 16 spermatids
(D) 32 spermatids

25. Head of sperm is formed from-
(A) nucleus of spermatid
(B) golgi apparatus of spermatid
(C) mitochondria of spermatid
(D) centrosome & centrioles of spermatid

26. Acrosomic cap of sperm is formed from-
(A) nucleus of spermatid
(B) golgi apparatus of spermatid
(C) mitochondria of spermatid
(D) centrosome & centrioles of spermatid

27. Axial filament & tail of sperm is formed from-
(A) nucleus of spermatid
(B) golgi apparatus of spermatid
(C) mitochondria of spermatid
(D) centrosome & centrioles of spermatid

28. Middle piece of sperm is formed from-
(A) nucleus of spermatid
(B) golgi apparatus of spermatid
(C) mitochondria of spermatid
(D) centrosome & centrioles of spermatid

29. Covering of sperm is formed from-
(A) endoplasmic retinaculum of spermatid
(B) cell membrane of spermatid
(C) mitochondria of spermatid
(D) centrosome & centrioles of spermatid

30. Axial filament of sperm is formed from-
(A) nucleus of spermatid
(B) golgi apparatus of spermatid
(C) mitochondria of spermatid
(D) anterior centrioles of spermatid

31. Spermatogenesis is completed in-
(A) 35 days
(B) 67-74 days
(C) 90 days
(D) 110-120 days

32. Type of respiration in the sperm is -
(A) aerobic
(B) anaerobic
(C) no respiration
(D) aerobic & anaerobic both

33. Sperm become motile after -
(A) full maturation
(B) mixing secretions of accessory sex glands
(C) since its formation
(D) none of the above

34. Sperms are having a capacity to fertilize an ovum up to-
(A) 24 hours (B) 48 hours
(C) 96 hours (D) one week

35. Length of fully mature sperm is-
(A) 24 microns (B) 50 microns
(C) 76 microns (D) 124 microns

Answer Sheet

1 (A)	2 (D)	3 (A)	4 (D)	5 (C)	6 (C)	7 (D)	8 (C)	9 (B)	10 (C)
11 (A)	12 (D)	13 (A)	14 (B)	15 (C)	16 (A)	17 (A)	18 (B)	19 (A)	20 (B)
21 (C)	22 (B)	23 (C)	24 (A)	25 (A)	26 (B)	27 (D)	28 (C)	29 (B)	30 (D)
31 (B)	32 (D)	33 (B)	34 (B)	35 (B)					

EXPLANATIONS

1. **(A)** The primordial sex cells (male and female) develop in the walls of yolk sac during 4th week of intra-uterine life. Then they migrate to come to lie inside developing gonad.
2. **(D)** A normal fertile male ejaculates about 3.5 ml of semen during intercourse containing about 250 million sperms (1 ml has 100 million sperms)
3. **(A)** The primordial germ cells migrate from the walls of yolk sac during 4th week of developmental life and enter gonad of genetically male. Here they remain dormant until puberty when hormonal changes in young male stimulate them to produce sperms.
4. **(D)** At birth, testis contains primordial germ cells that remain dormant till puberty (12 – 14 years). At puberty the spermatogonia divide and then differentiate into primary spermatocyte.
5. **(C)** The type B spermatogonia give rize to primary spermatocyte by undergoing DNA replication, thereby doubling the amount of DNA (2 x 2n= 4n) within the cell.
6. **(C)** The male hormone – testosterone is secreted by Leydig cells –129 interstitial cells of testis – the sertoli cells are the supporting cells. And Spermatogonia are responsible for production of sperms

7. D the head part of spermatozoan is formed by the nucleus of the spermatid. The mitochondria form the middle piece of spermatozoon. The centrioles occupy the two ends of middle piece.

Chapter 3

Female Sex Gland - Ovaries Öogenesis and Menstrual Cycle

1. During ovulation, the secondary oocyte remain at what specific stage of meiosis-
   (A) Prophase of meiosis I
   (B) Prophase of meiosis II
   (C) Metaphase of meiosis II
   (D) Metaphase of meiosis I

2. In production of female gamete, which of the following cells remain dormant for 12 – 40 years?
   (A) Primordial germ cells
   (B) Primary oocyte
   (C) Secondary oocyte
   (D) First polar body

3. A young woman has approximately 40,000 primary oocytes in her ovary at puberty. How many primary oocytes will be ovulated during entire reproductive life of women-
   (A) 40,000
   (B) 35,000
   (C) 480
   (D) 48

4. All primary oocytes are formed by-
   (A) 4th week of intra-uterine life
   (B) 5th month of intra-uterine life
   (C) At birth
   (D) At puberty

5. During maturation of female gamete (Oogenesis) when the oogonia undergo DNA replication in meiosis I to form primary oocyte-
   (A) During foetal life of 5th month
   (B) At birth
   (C) At puberty
   (D) With each ovarian cycle

6. In Oogenesis which event takes place immediately after completion of meiosis II-
   (A) Degeneration of zona pellucida
   (B) Sperm penetration of corona radiata
   (C) Formation of female pronucleus
   (D) Completion of cleavage

7. When does secondary oocyte complete its second meiotic division -
(A) At ovulation
(B) At fertilisation
(C) Before ovulation
(D) Before birth

8. Germinal epithelium of the ovary is-
(A) simple squamous
(B) simple cuboidal
(C) stratified cuboidal
(D) columnar ciliated

9. Oocytes present in the ovary at the time of birth –
(A) 4,00,000
(B) 40,000
(C) 4000
(D) 400

10. Ovum ovulated by female in her reproductive life is –
(A) 4,00,000
(B) 40,000
(C) 4000
(D) 400

11. Zona pellucida is seen in-
(A) primordial follicle
(B) primary follicle
(C) secondary follicle
(D) graffian follicle

12. Central oocyte with single layer of follicular cells is seen in-
(A) primordial follicle
(B) primary follicle
(C) secondary follicle
(D) graffian follicle

13. Zona pellucida, stratified cuboidal layers of granulosa cells and multiple golgi complexes are feature of –
(A) primordial follicle
(B) primary follicle
(C) secondary follicle
(D) graffian follicle

14. Oocyte surrounded by 6 to 12 layers of granulosa cells and antral space are feature of –
(A) primordial follicle
(B) primary follicle
(C) secondary follicle
(D) graffian follicle

15. Ovulation or release of ovum takes place from –
(A) primordial follicle
(B) primary follicle
(C) secondary follicle
(D) graffian follicle

16. Estrogen is secreted from-
(A) germinal epithelium
(B) theca interna
(C) theca externa
(D) corpus luteum

17. Ovulation takes place on –
(A) 7th day of menstrual cycle
(B) 10th day of menstrual cycle
(C) 14th day of menstrual cycle
(D) 21st day of menstrual cycle

18. Granulosa lutein cells secrete –
(A) estrogen
(B) progesterone
(C) follicle stimulating hormone
(D) luteinising hormone

19. Primary oocyte forms-
(A) 1 ovum
(B) 4 ova
(C) 8 ova
(D) 16 ova

20. Primary spermatocyte forms-
(A) 1 spermatozoa
(B) 4 spermatozoa
(C) 8 spermatozoa
(D) 16 spermatozoa

21. In the ovum at the time of ovulation –
(A) first meiotic division is in progress
(B) second meiotic division is in progress
(C) second mitotic division is in progress
(D) none of the above

22. Second meiotic division of ovum is completed at-
(A) during graffian follicle
(B) during ovulation
(C) at the time of fertilization
(D) at the time of implantation

23. Secondary oocyte is about –
(A) 50 μm
(B) 75 μm
(C) 150 μm
(D) 250 μm

24. Second polar body is seen in-
(A) perivitelline space
(B) inside the zona pellucida
(C) inside the secondary oocyte
(D) outside the zona pellucida

25. Ovum or secondary oocyte remains viable up to-
(A) 12-24 hours
(B) 24-48 hours
(C) 48-96 hours
(D) one week

26. Saw toothed uterine glands are seen in-
(A) follicular phase
(B) secretory phase
(C) menstrual phase
(D) all of the above

27. Spiral arteries in uterus are seen in –
(A) follicular phase
(B) secretory phase
(C) menstrual phase
(D) all of the above

28. Menstruation is caused by –
(A) increased estrogen & decreased progesterone
(B) increased estrogen & increased progesterone
(C) decreased estrogen & decreased progesterone
(D) decreased estrogen & increased progesterone

29. Ovulation takes place due to –
(A) high concentration of FSH
(B) high concentration of LH
(C) high concentration of estrogen
(D) high concentration of progesterone

30. Corpus luteum of menstruation remains functional till-
(A) One week
(B) two weeks
(C) one month
(D) none of the above

31. Corpus luteum of pregnancy remains functional till-
(A) two months
(B) three to four months
(C) five months
(D) nine months

32. True about the Ovum is –
(A) ova has 22+X CHROMOSOMES
(B) immotile cell
(C) large amount of cytoplasm
(D) all of the above

Answer Sheet

1 (C)	2 (B)	3 (C)	4 (B)	5 (A)	6 (C)	7 (B)	8 (B)	9 (A)	10 (D)
11 (B)	12 (A)	13 (B)	14 (C)	15 (D)	16 (B)	17 (C)	18 (B)	19 (A)	20 (B)
21 (B)	22 (C)	23 (C)	24 (A)	25 (A)	26 (A)	27 (B)	28 (C)	29 (A)	30 (B)
31 (B)	32 (D)								

EXPLANATIONS

1. **(C)** The secondary oocyte is arrested at metaphase of meiosis 11 about 3 hours before ovulation. It will remain in this stage until fertilisation occurs.
2. **(B)** Primary oocyte are formed in 5th month of foetal life and they remain dormant until puberty (12-14 years) when hormonal changes in young female stimulate ovarian and uterine cycle.
3. **(C)** During her reproductive life, a woman ovulates approximately 480 oocytes i.e (40 yer reproductive life x 12= 480 oocytes) provided she does not use oral contraceptions and become pregnant). The remaining oocytes disintegrates.
4. **(B)** All primary oocytes are formrd by 5th month of developmental life.At birth no oogonia are present, the female has her entire supply of primary oocyte to carry her through reproductive life.
5. **(C)** After meiosis 11 the secondary oocyte is arrested in metaphase and will remain in this stage till fertilisation occurs. Then secondary oocyte completes meosis 11, becomes mature ovum and sheds second polar body. The nucleus of mature ovum becomes female pronucleus.
6. **(B)** The secondary oocyte completes its second meiotic division at time of fertilisation, when it evicts the second polar body.

Chapter 4

Fertilisation, Early Development Of Embryo and Implantation

1. Where does the fertilisation takes place normally-
   (A) Inside vagina
   (B) Inside cervix of uterus
   (C) Inside ampulla of uterine tube
   (D) Near ovary

2. What are the processes that spermatozoa must undergo before entering the oocyte -
   (A) Capacitation
   (B) Acrosome reaction
   (C) Shedding of tail
   (D) Capacitation and acrosome reaction only

3. What is the viability of oocyte after ovulation without fertilisation -
   (A) 8 hours
   (B) 12 hours
   (C) 24 hours
   (D) 36 hours

4. All are the result of fertilisation except-
   (A) Restoration of diploid number of chromosomes
   (B) Determination of sex of embryo
   (C) Initiation of cleavage
   (D) Implantation of zygote

5. How soon after fertilisation the blastocyst begins implantation-
   (A) By 12 hours
   (B) By day 1
   (C) By day 4
   (D) By day 7

6. Where does blastocyst normally implant?
   (A) Functional layer of endometrium
   (B) Basal layer of endometrium
   (C) Myometrium
   (D) Perimetrium

7. Which of the following structures must degenerate for implantation of blastocysts to take place-
   (A) Endometrium in secretory phase
   (B) Zona pellucida
   (C) Synctiotrophoblast
   (D) Cytotrophoblast

8. What is the normal site of implantation of zygote?
   (A) Upper part posterior wall body of uterus
   (B) Lower part body of uterus
   (C) Uterine tube ampullary part
   (D) Cervix of uterus

9. The process of gastrulation of embryo includes all except-
   (A) Formation of primitive streak
   (B) Development of intra-embryonic mesoderm
   (C) Development of gut
   (D) Formation of trilaminar embryo

10. The chorion includes all three layer of developing embryo except-
   (A) Ectoderm
   (B) Parietal extra-embryonic mesoderm
   (C) Synctiotrophoblast
   (D) Cytotrophoblast

11. What are the remnants of notochord in an adult?
   (A) Nucleus pulposus of intervertebral discs
   (B) Ribs
   (C) Apical ligament of dens
   (D) A & C both

12. Time taken by oocyte to reach uterine lumen is-
   (A) one day
   (B) two day
   (C) three-four days
   (D) one week

13. Capacitation in the sperms takes about-
   (A) 7 minutes
   (B) 7 hours
   (C) 70 hours
   (D) 7 days

14. Acrosomic reaction has following processes except-
   (A) penetration of corona radiata
   (B) penetration of zona pellucida
   (C) capacitation
   (D) fusion of sperm & oocyte

15. Changes in ovum at the time of fertilization are-
   (A) second meiotic division is completed
   (B) second polar body is extruded
   (C) plasma membrane of oocyte & sperm unite
   (D) all of the above

16. Male pronucleus during fertilization is formed by-
   (A) sperm
   (B) head of the sperm
   (C) head & middle piece of sperm
   (D) middle piece & tail piece of sperm

17. After fertilization embryo reaches into-
   (A) one cell stage
   (B) two cell stage
   (C) four cell stage
   (D) none of the above

18. Outcome of fertilization is-
   (A) restoration of diploid number of chromosomes
   (B) sex determination
   (C) initiation of cleavage
   (D) all of the above

19. Changes taking place in first week of development are-
   (A) fertilization
   (B) implantation of blastocyst
   (C) formation of morula
   (D) all of the above

20. Blastomeres are formed from-
(A) primary oocyte
(B) secondary oocyte
(C) fertilized ovum
(D) unfertilized ovum

21. Embryo proper develops from-
(A) inner cell mass
(B) outer cell mass
(C) zona pellucida
(D) all of the above

22. Placenta develops from-
(A) inner cell mass
(B) outer cell mass/trophoblasts
(C) zona pellucida
(D) all of the above

23. For implantation of blastocyst most important step is-
(A) disappearance of zona pellucida
(B) epithelial wall of blastocyst
(C) formation of cavity
(D) all of the above

24. Animal pole of the blastocyst is-
(A) opposite to inner cell mass
(B) at the inner cell mass
(C) no such pole exists
(D) implanted site is called animal pole

25. Embryo is two celled at the age of-
(A) 2 days
(B) 4 days
(C) 8 days
(D) 16 days

26. Morula is formed at the age of-
(A) 2 days
(B) 3 days
(C) 4 days
(D) 8 days

27. Blastocyst is formed at the age of-
(A) 2 days
(B) 4 days
(C) 8 days
(D) 12 days

28. Blastocyst is embedded in endometrium on -
(A) 2 days
(B) 4 days
(C) 8 days
(D) 12 days

29. Embryonic bilaminar disc is formed at the age of-
(A) 2 days
(B) 4 days
(C) 8 days
(D) 12 days

30. Prochordal plate & primitive streak is formed at the age of-
(A) 8 days
(B) 14 days
(C) 18 days
(D) 24 days

31. Intra-embryonic mesoderm is formed at the age of-
(A) 32 days
(B) 16 days
(C) 12 days
(D) 8 days

32. Trilaminar disc or all three germ layers are formed at the age of-
(A) 32 days
(B) 16 days
(C) 12 days
(D) 8 days

33. Intra-embryonic ectoderm & endoderm is formed at the age of-
(A) 32 days
(B) 16 days
(C) 12 days
(D) 8 days

34. Pre-organogenesis period is-
(A) first week of pregnancy
(B) first two weeks of pregnancy
(C) first month of pregnancy
(D) none of the above

35. Embryonic period is-
(A) first two weeks of pregnancy
(B) first month of pregnancy
(C) third week to eighth week of pregnancy
(D) none of the above

36. First germ layer to be formed is-
(A) ectoderm
(B) mesoderm
(C) endoderm
(D) all are formed simultaneously

37. Second germ layer to be formed is-
(A) ectoderm
(B) mesoderm
(C) endoderm
(D) all are formed simultaneously

38. Flat cells of bilaminar embryo form-
(A) ectoderm
(B) mesoderm
(C) endoderm
(D) none of the above

39. Columnar cells of bilaminar embryo form-
(A) ectoderm
(B) mesoderm
(C) endoderm
(D) none of the above

40. Heuser's membrane lines the –
(A) amniotic cavity
(B) primary yolk sac
(C) maternal surface of placenta
(D) foetal surface of placenta

41. In bilaminar embryo roof of amniotic cavity is lined by trophoblasts while floor is formed by –
(A) endodermal flat cells
(B) ectodermal columnar cells
(C) mesodermal layer
(D) none of the above

42. Connecting stalk of embryo is formed by-
(A) ectoderm
(B) extra embryonic mesoderm
(C) endoderm
(D) mesoderm

43. With appearance of extra embryonic coelom the yolk sac becomes smaller and called secondary yolk sac is lined with-
(A) flat cells
(B) cuboidal cells
(C) columnar cells
(D) all of the above

44. Prochordal plate is developed in bilaminar disc-
(A) defines central axis
(B) right & left halves are defined
(C) head & tail ends are defined
(D) all of the above

45. Prochordal plate is developed in bilaminar disc from -
(A) upper ectodermal layer
(B) lower endodermal layer
(C) both A & B
(D) none of the above

46. Change noted in formation of prochordal plate is-
(A) columnar cells change into cuboidal
(B) cuboidal cells change into columnar
(C) columnar cells change into flat cells
(D) all of the above

47. Gastrulation phase is composed of –
(A) primitive streak formation
(B) formation of intraembryonic mesoderm
(C) both A & B
(D) none of the above

48. Primitive streak is formed from the tail end of prochordal plate by-
(A) endodermal cells
(B) mesodermal cells
(C) ectodermal cells
(D) all of the above

49. After formation of trilaminar embryo area which remains bilaminar is-
(A) buccopharyngeal membrane
(B) cloacal membrane
(C) both A & B
(D) all of the above

50. In ectopic pregnancy, implantation of blastocyst may take place in –
(A) uterine tube of uterus
(B) ovary
(C) peritoneal cavity
(D) all of the above

51. Epiblast layer of Embryonic disc forms–
(A) endoderm
(B) mesoderm
(C) ectoderm
(D) all of the above

52. Hypoblast layer of Embryonic disc forms –
(A) yolk sac
(B) mesoderm
(C) ectoderm
(D) endoderm

53. Amniotic sac develops on-
(A) endodermal side
(B) mesodermal side
(C) ectodermal side
(D) none of the above

54. Yolk sac develops on-
(A) endodermal side
(B) mesodermal side
(C) ectodermal side
(D) none of the above

55. During fertilization part of sperm that remains outside of the ovum-
(A) head of the sperm
(B) tail of the sperm
(C) plasma membrane of sperm
(D) none of the above

56. Acrosomal reaction at zona pellucida is caused by-
(A) lysosomal enzymes
(B) glycoproteins
(C) both A & B
(D) none of the above

57. Zona reaction at zona pellucida is caused by-
(A) lysosomal enzymes
(B) glycoproteins
(C) both A & B
(D) none of the above

58. Result of the fertilization between sperm and ovum –
(A) restoration of diploid number of chromosome
(B) cleavage formation
(C) sex determination of offspring
(D) all of the above

59. During test tube baby ovum is implanted in uterus at –
(A) two cell stage
(B) four cell stage
(C) eight cell stage
(D) sixteen cell stage

60. Test tube baby or in vitro fertilization is indicated in –
(A) sperm count less than 20000 per ml
(B) absence of ovulation
(C) tubal obstruction
(D) all of the above

61. Morula during cleavage is having –
(A) 16 cell stage
(B) 8 cell stage
(C) 4 cell stage
(D) none of the above

62. Extra embryonic mesoderm give rise to-
(A) musculoskeletal tissue
(B) connective tissue
(C) no tissue formation
(D) A & B both

63. Heuser's membrane line which cavity-
(A) amniotic cavity
(B) chorionic cavity
(C) primary yolk sac
(D) all of the above

64. In buccopharyngeal membrane which germ layer is absent-
(A) endoderm
(B) mesoderm
(C) ectoderm
(D) all are present

Answer Sheet

1 (C)	2 (D)	3 (C)	4 (D)	5 (D)	6 (A)	7 (B)	8 (A)	9 (C)	10 (C)
11 (D)	12 (C)	13 (B)	14 (C)	15 (D)	16 (B)	17 (B)	18 (D)	19 (D)	20 (C)
21 (A)	22 (B)	23 (A)	24 (B)	25 (A)	26 (B)	27 (B)	28 (C)	29 (C)	30 (B)
31 (B)	32 (B)	33 (D)	34 (B)	35 (C)	36 (C)	37 (A)	38 (C)	39 (A)	40 (B)
41 (B)	42 (B)	43 (B)	44 (D)	45 (B)	46 (B)	47 (C)	48 (C)	49 (C)	50 (D)
51 (D)	52 (A)	53 (C)	54 (A)	55 (C)	56 (B)	57 (A)	58 (D)	59 (C)	60 (D)
61 (A)	62 (C)	63 (C)	64 (B)						

EXPLANATIONS

1. (C) The fertilisation take place normally in the ampullary part of uterine tube
2. (D) The sperm has to undergo two processes capacitation (a process of conditioning of sperm in female genital tract that takes about 7 hours) and acrosome reaction (release of enzymes needed to penetrate zona pellucida)
3. (C) The oocyte that is shed after ovulation and is not fertilised, remains viable only for a period of 24 hours. After that it undergoes regression.
4. (D) The result of fertilisation are restoration of diploid number of chromosomes, determination of sex embryo and initiation of cleavage.
5. (D) The blastocyst begins the process of implantation in endometrium of uterus on 7th day after fertilisation.
6. (A) The blastocyst implants in functional layer of uterine endometrium. The basal layer is retained and serves as a source of regeneration of functional layer. The functional layer gets enlarged and more vascular for implantation.
7. (B) The zona pellucida must degenerate for implantation to occur. In early stage of cleavage of blastocyst, the blastomeres are surrounded by zona pellucida, the prevents implantation in uterine tube.
8. (A) The normal site of implantation of blastocysts is upper part posterior wall cavity of body of uterus. Other sites are known as abnormal sites of implantation.
9. (C) The process of gastrulation of embryo includes formation of primitive streak, development of intra- embryonic coelom and formation of trilaminar embryo.
11. (D) The remnants of notochord in adults are nucleus pulposus of intervertebral discs and apical ligament of dens

Chapter 5

Placenta Fetal Membranes Birth Defects and Twining

1. The intervillous spaces of placenta contain-
   (A) Maternal blood
   (B) Foetal blood
   (C) Amniotic blood
   (D) Maternal and foetal blood both

2. What is the normal amount of amniotic fluid at full term-
   (A) 50 ml
   (B) 500 ml
   (C) 1000 ml
   (D) 2000 ml

3. Which of the following structure does not pass through umbilical ring-
   (A) Allantois
   (B) Amnion
   (C) Yolk sac
   (D) Connecting stalk

4. The maternal and foetal components of placenta are-
   (A) Decidua, capsularis and secondary chorionic villi
   (B) Decidua, basalis and secondary chorionic villi
   (C) Decidua, parietalis and tertiary chorionic villi
   (D) Decidua, basalis and villous chorion

5. Which of the following best describe the placental components of dizygotic twins-
   (A) One placenta, two amniotic sac, one chorion
   (B) The placenta, two amniotic sac, two chorion
   (C) Two placenta, two amniotic sac, two chorion
   (D) One placenta, two amniotic sac, two chorion

6. The placental membrane that separates foetal and maternal blood in later stages of pregnancy consists of-
   (A) Synctiotrophoblast only
   (B) Cytotrophoblast only
   (C) Synctiotrophoblast and foetal endothelium
   (D) Synctiotrophoblast and cytotrophoblast

7. What are the main factors that causes congenital anomalies-
(A) Genetic factors only
(B) Environmental factors
(C) Genetic and environmental factors both
(D) Unknown factors

8. The main functions of placenta are following except-
(A) Transport of nutrients and excretion of waste products
(B) Exchange of gases via blood
(C) Production of hormones
(D) Growth of embryo and foetus

9. In decidual reaction changes that happen are-
(A) enlargement of stromal cells
(B) store glycogen &lipids
(C) develop vacuoles
(D) all of the above

10. Portion of the decidua where placenta will be formed is –
(A) decidua basalis
(B) decidua capsularis
(C) decidua parietalis
(D) all of the above

11. Portion of the decidua that separate the embryo from uterine cavity is –
(A) decidua basalis
(B) decidua capsularis
(C) decidua parietalis
(D) all of the above

12. Portion of the decidua which lines the rest of uterine cavity except for embryo is–
(A) decidua basalis
(B) decidua capsularis
(C) decidua parietalis
(D) all of the above

13. Decidual plate is actually –
(A) decidua basalis
(B) decidua capsularis
(C) decidua parietalis
(D) all of the above

14. Villi at the embryonic pole disappear by-
(A) end of second month
(B) end of third month
(C) end of fourth month
(D) end of fifth month

15. Primary chorionic villi has a-
(A) central core of cytotrophoblast
(B) surrounded by synctiotrophoblast
(C) extra embryonic mesoderm
(D) A & B both

16. Secondary chorionic villi has a-
(A) middle layer by cytotrophoblast
(B) surrounded by synctiotrophoblast
(C) central core of extra embryonic mesoderm
(D) all of the above

17. Tertiary chorionic villi has a-
(A) primary villi and blood vessel
(B) secondary villi and blood vessels
(C) both A & B
(D) none of the above

18. Foetal blood circulates through –
(A) primary chorionic villi
(B) secondary chorionic villi
(C) tertiary chorionic villi
(D) all of the above

19. True about anchoring villi is –
(A) first to develop
(B) attached on foetal side to primary mesoderm
(C) attached to cytotrophoblasts on maternal side
(D) all of the above

20. Foetal surface of placenta is-
(A) lined by amnion
(B) covered by chorion
(C) no cotyledons and smooth surface
(D) all of the above

21. Chorion frondosum is term given when-
(A) chorionic villi on abembryonic pole
(B) chorionic villi at decidua basalis
(C) both A & B
(D) none of the above

22. Chorion levae is term given when-
(A) chorionic villi on abembryonic pole
(B) chorionic villi at decidua basalis
(C) both A & B
(D) none of the above

23. Cavity which is enclosed in Heuser's membrane is-
(A) primary yolk sac
(B) secondary yolk sac
(C) tertiary yolk sac
(D) all of the above

24. Earliest blood vessels are noted in the-
(A) primary yolk sac
(B) secondary yolk sac
(C) tertiary yolk sac
(D) all of the above

25. Yolk sac which remains outside the embryo is-
(A) primary yolk sac
(B) secondary yolk sac
(C) tertiary yolk sac
(D) all of the above

26. Yolk sac which remains in communication with midgut through vitello intestinal duct is-
(A) primary yolk sac
(B) secondary yolk sac
(C) tertiary yolk sac
(D) all of the above

27. Which one of the following is ectodermal in origin-
(A) amnion
(B) yolk sac
(C) allantois
(D) all of the above

28. Definitive yolk sac is –
(A) primary yolk sac
(B) secondary yolk sac
(C) tertiary yolk sac
(D) all of the above

29. True about allantois is all except-
(A) endodermal diverticulum
(B) from the hind gut
(C) ectodermal diverticulum
(D) give rise to cloaca

30. Events part of the decidual reaction is-
(A) stromal cells enlarge
(B) store glycogen & lipids
(C) become vacuolated
(D) all of the above

31. Cytotrophoblasts & syncytiotrophoblasts are differentiated from trophoblasts on-
(A) 7th day
(B) 8th day
(C) 11th day
(D) 16th day

32. Lacunar space appear in the syncytium on-
(A) 7th day
(B) 8th day
(C) 9th day
(D) 16th day

33. Embryo gets completely implanted in endometrium on-
(A) 7th day
(B) 8th day
(C) 9th day
(D) 11th day

34. Primary villi are formed on-
(A) 11th day
(B) 13th day
(C) 18th day
(D) 24th day

35. Secondary & tertiary villi are formed on-
(A) 11th day
(B) 13th day
(C) 16th day
(D) 24th day

36. Villi are seen all around the trophoblasts-
(A) 24th day
(B) 30th day
(C) 2nd month
(D) 4th month

37. Definitive placenta is formed on-
(A) 2nd month
(B) 3rd month
(C) 4th month
(D) 5th month

Answer Sheet

1 (A)	2 (C)	3 (B)	4 (D)	5 (D)	6 (C)	7 (C)	8 (D)	9 (D)	10 (A)
11 (B)	12 (C)	13 (A)	14 (B)	15 (D)	16 (D)	17 (B)	18 (C)	19 (D)	20 (D)
21 (B)	22 (A)	23 (A)	24 (B)	25 (C)	26 (C)	27 (A)	28 (C)	29 (C)	30 (D)
31 (B)	32 (C)	33 (D)	34 (B)	35 (C)	36 (C)	37 (C)			

EXPLANATIONS

1. **(A)** The intervillous spaces of placenta are filled with maternal blood. The foetal blood lies in the foetal blood vessels contained in chorionic villi. The amniotic fluid fills up the amniotic sac that surrounds the developing embryo and foetus.
2. **(C)** The normal amount of amniotic fluid at full term is 1000 ml. Oligohydramnios (400 ml) in late pregnancy is indicative of renal agenesis. Polyhydramnios (2000 ml) in late pregnancy is indicative of anencephaly.
3. **(B)** The amnion does not pass through umbilical ring. As the head and tail folds of embryo occur the amnion becomes outer covering of umbilical cord.
4. **(D)** The placenta is a composites organ consisting of tissue from twp different source- the mother and foetus. The maternal component is decidua basalis and foetal component is villous chorion.
5. **(D)** The dizygotic twins and 35% of monozygotic twins have two placenta, two amniotic sacs and two chorion.

6. **(C)** During later stages of pregnancy, the placental membrane consists of syncitiotrophoblast and foetal endothelium.
7. **(C)** The main factors that cause congenital anamolies are both genetic factors and environmental factors. About 80% of all congenital anamolies are produced by combination of genetic and environmental factors. The remaining 20% -half are caused by genetic factors and other half by environmental factors only.
8. **(D)** The main functions of placenta are transport of nutrients and excretion of waste products, exchange of gases via blood and production of hormones. The placenta is not directly involved in growth of embryo and foetus.

Chapter 6

Pharyngeal Arches

1. What are the mesodermal derivatives of pharyngeal arches?
   (A) Muscle, skeletal element and aortic arch
   (B) Epithelium of mouth cavity
   (C) Salivary glands
   (D) Parathyroid glands

2. What are ectodermal derivatives of branchial arches?
   (A) Skin over lower jaw, and side of neck
   (B) Epidermal lining of external acoustic meatus
   (C) Outer cuticular layer of tympanic membrane
   (D) Cervical sinus that obliterates later on and may give rise to branchial cyst.
   (E) All of the above

3. What are endodermal derivatives of 4th pharyngeal pouch-
   (A) Parathyroid1V and caudal pharyngeal complex that gives rise to thymus, cells of thyroid and ultimo branchial body
   (B) Palatine tonsil
   (C) Parathyroid III
   (D) Thyroglossal duct

4. The most common site of thyroglossal cyst is-
   (A) Anterior border of sternomastoid
   (B) Superior mediastinum
   (C) Base of tongue
   (D) Midline close to hyoid bone

5. During surgery of removal of thyroid gland, a number of small masses of glandular tissue are noted just lateral to thyroid. What these masses can be-
   (A) Metastases from thyroid tumors
   (B) Ectopic glandular tissue belonging to thymus and parathyroid
   (C) Thyroglossal cysts
   (D) Ectopic parathyroid

6. Taste sensation from oral part(anterior two third) of tongue is predominantly carried by-
   (A) Trigeminal nerve
   (B) Glossopharyngeal nerve
   (C) Chorda tympani branch of facial nerve
   (D) Recurrent laryngeal branch of vagus nerve

7. The epithelium of tongue develops from-
(A) 1st, 3rd and 4th arch endoderm
(B) 1st arch endoderm
(C) 3rd arch endoderm
(D) 1st and 3rd arch endoderm

8. The muscles of tongue develops from-
(A) Pre-occipital myotomes
(B) Occipital myotomes
(C) Cervical myotomes
(D) Mesenchyme locally

9. Meckel's cartilage is cartilage of the –
(A) 1st branchial arch
(B) 2nd branchial arch
(C) 3rd branchial arch
(D) 6th branchial arch

10. Richter's cartilage is cartilage of-
(A) 1st branchial arch
(B) 2nd branchial arch
(C) 3rd branchial arch
(D) 6th branchial arch

11. Bones formed from the first branchial arch are all except–
(A) malleus
(B) incus
(C) stapes
(D) mandible

12. Ligaments derived from first branchial arch are-
(A) sphenomandibular ligament
(B) sphenomandibular ligament & anterior ligament of malleus
(C) sphenomandibular ligament & stylomandibular ligament
(D) sphenomandibular, stylomandibular & ant ligament of malleus

13. Bones developed from first branchial arch are-
(A) zygomatic bone
(B) palatine bone
(C) temporal bone
(D) ll of the above

14. Muscles derived from first branchial arch are all except-
(A) tensor tympani
(B) tensor veli palati
(C) digastric posterior belly
(D) temporalis

15. Nerve of the first branchial arch is-
(A) mandibular nerve & facial nerve
(B) mandibular nerve & chorda tympani nerve
(C) facial nerve & glossopharyngeal nerve
(D) facial nerve & lingual nerve

16. Nerve of the second branchial arch is-
(A) mandibular nerve
(B) chorda tympani nerve
(C) glossopharyngeal nerve
(D) facial nerve

17. Nerve of the third branchial arch is-
(A) facial nerve
(B) glossopharyngeal nerve
(C) vagus nerve
(D) lingual nerve

18. Nerve of the fourth branchial arch is-
(A) mandibular nerve
(B) facial nerve
(C) glossopharyngeal nerve
(D) superior laryngeal nerve

19. Nerve of the sixth branchial arch is-
(A) superior laryngeal nerve
(B) vagus nerve
(C) glossopharyngeal nerve
(D) recurrent laryngeal nerve

20. Nerve of the somitomere 1 & 2 is-
(A) optic nerve
(B) ophthalmic nerve
(C) occulomotor nerve
(D) trochlear nerve

21. Nerve of the somitomere 3 is-
(A) optic nerve
(B) ophthalmic nerve
(C) occulomotor nerve
(D) trochlear nerve

22. Nerve of the somitomere 4 is-
(A) mandibular nerve
(B) ophthalmic nerve
(C) occulomotor nerve
(D) trochlear nerve

23. Nerve of the somitomere 5 is-
(A) mandibular nerve
(B) facial nerve
(C) abduscence nerve
(D) trochlear nerve

24. Nerve of the somitomere 6 is-
(A) mandibular nerve
(B) abduscence nerve
(C) facial nerve
(D) glossopharyngeal nerve

25. Nerve of the somitomere 7 is-
(A) mandibular nerve
(B) facial nerve
(C) glossopharyngeal nerve
(D) vagus nerve

26. Nerve of the occipital somites 1 & 2 is-
(A) mandibular nerve
(B) facial nerve
(C) glossopharyngeal nerve
(D) vagus nerve

27. Nerve of the occipital somites 3-5 is-
(A) hypoglossal nerve
(B) facial nerve
(C) glossopharyngeal nerve
(D) vagus nerve

28. Stylopharyngeus muscle develops from-
(A) somitomere 5
(B) somitomere 6
(C) somitomere 7
(D) all of the above

29. First pharyngeal pouch give rise to-
(A) tongue
(B) auditory tube
(C) middle ear cavity
(D) all of the above

30. second pharyngeal pouch give rise to-
(A) palatine tonsil
(B) auditory tube
(C) middle ear cavity
(D) all of the above

31. Third pharyngeal pouch give rise to-
(A) superior parathyroid & thyroid
(B) inferior parathyroid & thyroid
(C) inferior parathyroid & thymus
(D) all of the above

32. Fourth pharyngeal pouch give rise to-
(A) superior parathyroid & thyroid
(B) inferior parathyroid & thyroid
(C) inferior parathyroid & thymus
(D) all of the above

33. True about caudal pharyngeal complex is-
(A) formed by ultimobranchial body of fifth & fourth arch
(B) parafollicular C cells are derived from it
(C) superior parathyroid gland develops from it
(D) all of the above

34. Which of the parathyroid is relatively fixed in its position-
(A) superior parathyroid
(B) inferior parathyroid
(C) both A & B
(D) none of the above

35. Ectopic thyroid tissue may be found in-
(A) pons
(B) larynx
(C) trachea
(D) all of the above

36. 1st & 2nd branchial arches are seen at the age –
(A) 4th week
(B) 5th week
(C) 6th week
(D) 7th week

37. Formation of thyroid gland is seen at the age of-
(A) 4th week
(B) 5th week
(C) 6th week
(D) 7th week

38. Formation of thymus & parathyroid gland is seen at the age of-
(A) 4th week
(B) 5th week
(C) 6th week
(D) 7th week

39. Thyroid gland reaches it's definitive position in –
(A) 4th week
(B) 5th week
(C) 6th week
(D) 7th week

40. Artery of the first branchial arch is –
(A) maxillary artery
(B) lingual artery
(C) stapedial artery
(D) all of the above

41. Artery of the second branchial arch is–
(A) maxillary artery
(B) lingual artery
(C) stapedial artery
(D) all of the above

42. Artery of the third branchial arch is –
(A) maxillary artery
(B) lingual artery
(C) stapedial artery
(D) common & external carotid artery

43. Artery of the fourth branchial arch on right side is –
(A) maxillary artery
(B) lingual artery
(C) right subclavian artery
(D) all of the above

44. Artery of the fourth branchial arch on left side is –
(A) maxillary artery
(B) arch of aorta
(C) right subclavian artery
(D) all of the above

45. Artery of the sixth branchial arch on left side is –
(A) maxillary artery
(B) arch of aorta
(C) right subclavian artery
(D) pulmonary artery

Answer Sheet

1. (A)	2. (E)	3. (A)	4. (D)	5. (B)	6. (C)	7. (A)	8. (B)	9. (A)	10. (B)
11. (C)	12. (B)	13. (D)	14. (C)	15. (B)	16. (D)	17. (B)	18. (D)	19. (D)	20. (C)
21. (D)	22. (A)	23. (C)	24. (C)	25. (C)	26. (D)	27. (A)	28. (C)	29. (D)	30. (D)
31. (C)	32. (A)	33. (D)	34. (A)	35. (D)	36. (A)	37. (B)	38. (B)	39. (D)	40. (A)
41. (C)	42. (D)	43. (C)	44. (B)	45. (D)					

EXPLANATIONS

1. **(A)** The mesodermal derivatives of pharyngeal arches are muscle, skeletal element and an aortic arch. The mixed nerve of the corresponding pharyngeal arch supplies the muscle.

2. **(E)** The ectodermal derivatives of branchial arches are skin over lower jaw and side of neck, the epidermal lining of external acoustic meatus, the outer cuticular lining of tympanic membrane and cervical sinus that obliterates later on, but may give rise to branchial cyst.

3. **(A)** The endodermal derivatives of 4th pharyngeal pouch are parathyroid IV (superior parathyroid) and caudal pharyngeal complex that gives rise to parafollicular cells (C cells) of thyroid gland and ultimo-branchial body.

4. **(D)** The most common site of thyroglossal cyst is midline close to hyoid bone. The thyroid gland develops from the thyroglossal duct that is formed in midline in floor of pharynx. The duct descends in midline passing ventral to hyoid bone to reach its adult position.

5. **(B)** Small masses of glandular tissue that are found just lateral to thyroid gland during surgery of thyroid gland are usually ectopic glandular tissue belonging to thymus gland or parathyroid gland.

6. **(C)** Taste sensation from oral part (anterior two third) of tongue is carried by chorda tympani of facial nerve. As this part of tongue is developed from endoderm of 1st pharyngeal arch the general sensation are carried by trigeminal nerve.

7. **(A)** The epithelium of tongue develops from 1st,3rd and 4th pharyngeal arches. The two lingual swellings and tuberculum impar is from 1st arch, while the hypo-branchial eminence (copula) from 3rd arch and 4th arch from the rest of epithelium. The 2nd arch is excluded.

8. **(B)** The muscles of tongue develop from occipital myotomes that migrate ventrally along epicardial ridge to come to lie in developing tongue. They also carry their nerve supply- hypoglossal nerve along with them.

Chapter 7

Face, Nose and Palate

1. What is the most common congenital malformation of head and neck region-
(A) Anterior cleft palate
(B) Posterior cleft palate
(C) Unilateral cleft palate
(D) Ankyloglossia

2. The inter -maxillary segment of palate is formed by fusion of-
(A) Palatine shelves
(B) Maxillary prominences
(C) Two medial nasal prominences
(D) Two lateral nasal prominences

3. The upper lip is formed by-
(A) Maxillary processes
(B) Fronto- nasal processes
(C) Maxillary processes and median nasal processes
(D) Median nasal processes

4. The external ear is formed by-
(A) 1st ectodermal cleft
(B) Tubercles growing on 1st and 2nd arches around 1st cleft
(C) Mesenchyme
(D) Ectoderm

5. Oblique facial cleft is formed by-
(A) Non –fusion of maxillary and lateral nasal process
(B) Fronto-nasal process
(C) Maxillary process
(D) Lateral nasal process

6. What is the most common site of a pharyngeal fistula-
(A) Dorsal aspect of neck
(B) Anterior border of sternomastoid
(C) Superior mediastinum
(D) Midline close to hyoid bone

7. Mesodermal basis of the lateral part of upper lip is from-
(A) mandibular process
(B) maxillary process
(C) median nasal process
(D) all of the above

8. Mesodermal basis of the median portion or philtrum of upper lip is from-
(A) mandibular process
(B) maxillary process
(C) median nasal process
(D) all of the above

9. Upper lip is formed by maxillary & frontonasal process, skin of the upper lip is supplied by the branches from-
(A) ophthalmic division of trigeminal nerve
(B) maxillary division of trigeminal nerve
(C) both A & B
(D) both A & B along with facial nerve

10. Upper lip is supplied by –
(A) maxillary nerve
(B) ophthalmic division of trigeminal nerve
(C) facial nerve
(D) A & C both

11. Cheeks are formed by the-
(A) maxillary process
(B) mandibular process
(C) frontonasal process
(D) both A & B

12. Nasolacrimal duct is formed at naso optic furrow and is-
(A) endodermal origin
(B) mesodermal origin
(C) ectodermal origin
(D) all of the above

13. Paranasal sinus developing before birth is –
(A) frontal
(B) sphenoid
(C) ethmoidal sinuses
(D) all of the above

14. Paranasal sinus developing before birth is –
(A) frontal
(B) maxillary
(C) ethmoidal sinuses
(D) all of the above

15. Primitive palate is extension of-
(A) maxillary process
(B) frontonasal process
(C) both A & B
(D) none of the above

16. Premaxilla bearing incisor teeth is an extension of-
(A) maxillary process
(B) frontonasal process
(C) both A & B
(D) none of the above

17. Lens placodes are seen at the age of-
(A) third week
(B) fourth week
(C) fifth week
(D) sixth week

18. Frontonasal, maxillary & mandibular processes are seen at the age of-
(A) third week
(B) fourth week
(C) fifth week
(D) sixth week

19. Nasal placodes are seen at the age of-
(A) third week
(B) fourth week
(C) fifth week
(D) sixth week

20. Nasal pits are seen at the age of-
(A) third week
(B) fourth week
(C) fifth week
(D) sixth week

21. Palatal processes of maxilla are seen at the age of-
(A) third week
(B) fourth week
(C) fifth week
(D) sixth week

22. Development of pinna is seen at the age of-
(A) third week
(B) fourth week
(C) fifth week
(D) sixth week

23. Eye lids are seen at the age of-
(A) fifth week
(B) sixth week
(C) seventh week
(D) eighth week

24. Fusion of maxillary palatal process along with frontonasal process is noted at the age of-
(A) fifth week
(B) sixth week
(C) seventh week
(D) eighth week

25. Eyes are shifted to frontal position from lateral position at the age of-
(A) fifth week
(B) sixth week
(C) seventh week
(D) eighth week

26. Bucconasal membrane ruptures at the age of-
(A) third week
(B) sixth week
(C) seventh week
(D) eighth week

27. Buccopharyngeal membrane ruptures at the age of-
(A) fourth week beginning
(B) sixth week
(C) seventh week
(D) eighth week

28. Palatal processes and nasal process fuse at the age of-
(A) seventh week
(B) eighth week
(C) ninth week
(D) tenth week

29. Teratogens most likely cause lip defects at the age of-
(A) third week
(B) fourth & fifth week
(C) fifth & sixth week
(D) seventh & eighth week

30. Teratogens most likely cause cleft palate defects at the age of-
(A) third week
(B) fourth & fifth week
(C) fifth & sixth week
(D) seventh & eighth week

Answer Sheet

1 (C)	2 (C)	3 (C)	4 (B)	5 (A)	6 (B)	7 (B)	8 (C)	9 (B)	10 (D)
11 (D)	12 (C)	13 (B)	14 (B)	15 (B)	16 (B)	17 (B)	18 (B)	19 (B)	20 (C)
21 (D)	22 (D)	23 (C)	24 (C)	25 (D)	26 (D)	27 (A)	28 (D)	29 (C)	30 (D)

EXPLANATIONS

1. **(C)** Unilateral cleft palate is the most common congenital anomaly of head and neck region. It occurs in about 1 to 900 births and may be unilateral or bilateral. Cleft lip occurs when maxillary process fail to fuse with medial nasal process
2. **(C)** The intermaxillary segment of palate that plays an important role in formation of definitive palate, is formed, when two medial nasal prominences fuse in the midline.
3. **(C)** According to most of the embryologists, the upper lip is bilateral in origin. It develops from fusion of maxillary process and median nasal process (that is called globular process)
4. **(B)** Pinna (external ear) is formed by sic tubercles growing at dorsal ends of 1st and 2nd arches around 1st ectodermal cleft. The tubercles consist of ectoderm with mesoderm inside.
5. **(A)** Oblique facial cleft is formed by non-fusion of maxillary and lateral nasal process between the eye and ala of nose. The fusion between these two processes leads to formation of an ectodermal groove that eventually forms lacrimal sacs and nasolacrimal duct.
6. **(B)** The most common site of pharyngeal fistula is along the anterior border of sternomastoid. The pharyngeal fistula forms when pharyngeal pouch 2 and ectodermal cleft 2 persist along the lateral aspect of neck.

Chapter 8

Respiratory System

1. What is the first sign of development of respiratory system?
   (A) Hypobranchial eminence
   (B) Respiratory diverticulum
   (C) Primitive foregut
   (D) Tracheo-oesophageal fistula

2. The trachea is lined by pseudo- stratified columnar epithelium with goblet cells. This epithelium is derived from-
   (A) Ectoderm
   (B) Endoderm
   (C) Visceral mesoderm
   (D) Mesoderm of 4th and 6th pharyngeal pouches

3. Smooth muscle, connective tissue and cartilage of primary bronchi are derived from-
   (A) Ectoderm
   (B) Endoderm
   (C) Visceral mesoderm
   (D) Mesoderm of 4th and 6th branchial arches

4. Immediately after birth the baby has laboured breathing. It becomes cyanotic and dies. What can be the possible cause-
   (A) Congenital emphysema
   (B) Cystic fibrosis
   (C) Pulmonary carcinoma
   (D) Respiratory distress syndrome

5. The blood-air barrier in the lung consists of -
   (A) Ectoderm only
   (B) Visceral mesoderm only
   (C) Visceral mesoderm and ectoderm
   (D) Visceral mesoderm and endoderm

6. The thyroid, cricoid and arytenoids cartilage of larynx develop from -
   (A) Skeletal element of 1st branchial arches
   (B) Skeletal element of 4th and 6th branchial arches
   (C) Skeletal element of 2nd branchial arch
   (D) Skeletal element of 3rd branchial arch.

7. The respiratory diverticulum is initially an open communication with primitive gut. Which of the following embryonic structures is responsible for separating the two-
   (A) Laryngo-tracheal diverticulum
   (B) Laryngo-tracheal groove
   (C) Tracheo-oesophageal/septum
   (D) Bronchio-pulmonary segment

8. Thyroid, cricoid & arytenoid cartilages develop from –
(A) 4th branchial arch
(B) 6th branchial arch
(C) 4th & 6th branchial arch
(D) Hypobranchial eminence

9. Respiratory diverticulum appears at the age of –
(A) fourth week
(B) fifth week
(C) sixth week
(D) seventh week

10. Epiglottis develops from –
(A) 4th branchial arch
(B) 6th branchial arch
(C) 4th & 6th branchial arch
(D) Hypobranchial eminence

11. Number of lobar bronchi before birth is-
(A) about 11
(B) about 17
(C) about 23
(D) about 28

12. Number of lobar bronchi after birth is-
(A) about 11
(B) about 17
(C) about 23
(D) about 28

13. During foetal life bronchial tree and subdivisions are lined with-
(A) cuboidal epithelium
(B) columnar epithelium
(C) pseudostratified epithelium
(D) all of the above

14. Lung buds appear at the age of-
(A) fourth week
(B) fifth week
(C) sixth week
(D) seventh week

15. Pseudo glandular period of maturation of lungs is-
(A) 5-16 weeks
(B) 16-26 weeks
(C) 26 weeks - birth
(D) 8th month – childhood

16. Canalicular period of maturation of lungs is-
(A) 5-16 weeks
(B) 16-26 weeks
(C) 26 weeks - birth
(D) 8th month – childhood

17. Terminal sac period of maturation of lungs is-
(A) 5-16 weeks
(B) 16-26 weeks
(C) 26 weeks - birth
(D) 8th month – childhood

18. Alveolar period of maturation of lungs is-
(A) 5-16 weeks
(B) 16-26 weeks
(C) 26 weeks - birth
(D) 8th month – childhood

19. Surfactant is secreted by-
(A) type I alveolar epithelial cells
(B) type II alveolar epithelial cells
(C) both A & B
(D) none of the above

20. Type II alveolar epithelial cells are developing at the age of-
(A) 5th month of intrauterine life
(B) 6th month of intrauterine life
(C) 7th month of intrauterine life
(D) 8th month of intrauterine life

21. Alveoli present at the birth are-
(A) 1/6th of adult
(B) 1/4th of adult
(C) 1/3rd of adult
(D) half of the adult

22. Premature infant is able to survive at the age of-
(A) 5th month
(B) 6th month
(C) 7th month
(D) 8th month

23. Alveoli reach to the adult status by the age of –
(A) third year
(B) sixth year
(C) tenth year
(D) puberty

Answer Sheet

1 (B)	2 (B)	3 (C)	4 (D)	5 (D)	6 (B)	7 (C)	8 (C)	9 (A)	10 (D)
11 (B)	12 (C)	13 (A)	14 (B)	15 (A)	16 (B)	17 (C)	18 (D)	19 (B)	20 (B)
21 (A)	22 (C)	23 (C)							

EXPLANATIONS

1 **(B)** The first sign of development of respiratory system is formation of respiratory diverticulum from caudal end of primitive pharynx.

2 **(B)** The pseudo-stratified columnar epithelium with goblet cells of trachea is derived from endoderm. The epithelium lining of entire respiratory passage and up to alveoli is from visceral endoderm.

3 **(C)** The smooth muscle' connective tissue and cartilage of primary bronchi are derived from visceral mesoderm.

4 **(D)** Respiratory distress syndrome is common in premature infants and infants of diabetic mothers. It is caused by deficiency of or absence of surfactant. Collapsed alveoli and collection of eosinophilic material can be observed histologically.

5 **(D)** The blood-air barrier in the lung consists of visceral mesoderm and endoderm. The visceral mesoderm forms the epithelial lining of blood capillaries and endoderm forms the lining of alveoli.

6 **(B)** The thyroid, cricoid and arytenoid cartilage develop from skeletal elements of 4th and 6th branchial arches.

7 **(C)** When Tracheo-oesophageal folds fuse in midline they form trachea-oesophageal septum. This septum is responsible for separating adult trachea ventrally from oesophagus dorsally.

Chapter **9**

Nervous System

1. The anterior and posterior neuropore of developing neural tubes close during-
(A) 2nd week of development
(B) 4th week of development
(C) 5th week of development
(D) 6th week of development

2. Third ventricle is the cavity of which part of brain-
(A) Telencephalon
(B) Mesencephalon
(C) Diencephalon
(D) Rhombocephalon

3. Which of the following structure develops from diencephalon-
(A) Caudate nucleus
(B) Cerebellum
(C) Adenohypophysis
(D) Neurohypophysis

4. At birth conus medullaris of spinal cord lies at which level-
(A) T12
(B) L1
(C) L3
(D) L2

5. Which of the following nucleus represents the general somatic efferent column of pons-
(A) Abducent nucleus
(B) Nucleus ambiguous
(C) Hypoglossal nucleus
(D) Inferior olivary nucleus

6. Which of the following nucleus represents the special visceral efferent column in medulla oblongata?
(A) Dorsal nucleus of Vegas
(B) Hypoglossal nucleus
(C) Nucleus ambiguous
(D) Inferior vestibular nucleus

7. Which of the following structure is derived from telencephalon-
(A) Pineal gland
(B) Hippocampus
(C) Hypothalamus
(D) Optic nerve

8. The flexure that develops between the metencephalon and mylencephalon is called-
(A) Cephalic flexure
(B) Mesencephalic flexure
(C) Cerebellar flexure
(D) Pontine flexure

9. Which of the following statement best describe the sulcus limitans-
(A) Found in interpenduncular fossa
(B) Separates medulla and pons
(C) Separates alar and basal lamina
(D) Separates hypothalamus and thalamus

10. Which of the following condition describes herniation of meninges and spinal cord through a defect in vertebrae-
(A) Spina bifida with meningomyelocele
(B) Spina bifida with meningocele
(C) Spina bifida with myelocele
(D) Arnold Chiari Syndrome

11. Cerebellum develops from-
(A) Diencephalon
(B) Rhombic lip of alar lamina
(C) Basal lamina
(D) Mylencephalon

12. The choroid plexus of fourth ventricle is derived from-
(A) Alar plate
(B) Basal plate
(C) Roof plate
(D) Floor plate

13. Myelinated preganglionic sympathetic neurons have their cell bodies in-
(A) Clark's column
(B) Substantia gelatinosa
(C) Posterior grey column
(D) Intermediate lateral cell column

14. Which structure is derived from cranial neural crest cells -
(A) Piamater
(B) Lens of eyeball
(C) Duramater
(D) Pineal gland

15. Neural plate appears at the beginning of –
(A) two weeks
(B) three weeks
(C) four weeks
(D) five weeks

16. Formation of neural tube begins in the–
(A) cervical region
(B) thoracic region
(C) lumbar region
(D) sacral region

17. Closure of the cranial neuropore takes on-
(A) 21st day
(B) 23rd day
(C) 25th day
(D) 32nd day

18. Closure of the caudal neuropore takes on-
(A) 21st day
(B) 23rd day
(C) 25th day
(D) 27th day

19. Closure of the cranial neuropore takes on-
(A) 16-20 somite stage
(B) 18-20 somite stage
(C) 22-25 somite stage
(D) 27th somite stage

20. Cervical flexure during developing central nervous system appears –
(A) junction between hind brain & spinal cord
(B) junction between hind brain & mid brain
(C) junction between mid-brain & spinal cord
(D) within midbrain

21. Cephalic flexure during developing central nervous system appears –
(A) junction between hind brain & spinal cord
(B) junction between hind brain & mid brain
(C) junction between mid-brain & spinal cord
(D) within midbrain

22. Pontine flexure during developing central nervous system appears –
(A) junction between hind brain & spinal cord
(B) junction between metencephalon & myelencephalon
(C) junction between telencephalon & prosencephalon
(D) within midbrain

23. Telencephalic flexure during developing central nervous system appears –
(A) junction between hind brain & spinal cord
(B) junction between telencephalon & prosencephalon
(C) junction between metencephalon & myelencephalon
(D) within midbrain

24. Parts of brain derived from Rhombocephalon are –
(A) pons
(B) cerebellum
(C) medulla
(D) all of the above

25. All are derived from diencephalon except-
(A) adenohypophysis
(B) neurohypophysis
(C) thalamus
(D) hypothalamus

26. Parts of brain derived from myelencephalon are –
(A) pons
(B) cerebellum
(C) medulla
(D) spinal cord

27. Pons develops from the –
(A) myelencephalon
(B) metencephalon
(C) telencephalon
(D) rhombic lip

28. Fourth ventricle is the cavity of –
(A) prosencephalon
(B) mesencephalon
(C) rhombocephalon
(D) none of the above

29. Third ventricle is the cavity of –
(A) prosencephalon
(B) mesencephalon
(C) rhombocephalon
(D) none of the above

30. Lateral ventricle is the cavity of –
(A) prosencephalon
(B) mesencephalon
(C) rhombocephalon
(D) none of the above

31. Cerebral aqueduct is the cavity of –
(A) prosencephalon
(B) mesencephalon
(C) rhombocephalon
(D) none of the above

32. Neuroepithelial cells in the developing brain –
(A) pseudostratified epithelium
(B) seen after closure of neural pore
(C) they form neuroblasts
(D) all are true

33. Mantle layer of the neural tube forms-
(A) white matter of spinal cord
(B) grey matter of spinal cord
(C) both A & C
(D) none of the above

34. Marginal layer of the neural tube forms-
(A) white matter of spinal cord
(B) grey matter of spinal cord
(C) both A & C
(D) none of the above

35. First cell which develops from neuroblasts is-
(A) apolar neuroblast
(B) unipolar neuroblast
(C) bipolar neuroblast
(D) multipolar neuroblast

36. Unipolar neuroblast which develops from primitive neuroblasts is then converted into-
(A) apolar neuroblast
(B) unipolar neuroblast
(C) bipolar neuroblast
(D) multipolar neuroblast

37. Apolar neuroblast which develops from primitive neuroblasts is then converted into-
(A) apolar neuroblast
(B) unipolar neuroblast
(C) bipolar neuroblast
(D) multipolar neuroblast

38. Multipolar neuroblast is transformation of-
(A) apolar neuron neuroblast
(B) unipolar neuroblast
(C) bipolar neuroblast
(D) multipolar neuroblast

39. Gliablasts are derived from the –
(A) primitive neuroepithelial cells of neural tube
(B) neural crest
(C) mesenchyme
(D) all of the above

40. Astrocytes are derived from the –
(A) primitive neuroepithelial cells of neural tube
(B) neural crest
(C) mesenchyme
(D) all of the above

41. Microglial cells are derived from the –
(A) primitive neuroepithelial cells of neural tube
(B) neural crest
(C) mesenchyme
(D) all of the above

42. Oligodendrocytes are primarily seen in-
(A) mantle layer
(B) marginal layer
(C) both A & B
(D) none of the above

43. Astrocytes are primarily seen in-
(A) mantle layer
(B) marginal layer
(C) both A & B
(D) none of the above

44. Myelin sheath is formed by –
(A) astrocytes
(B) oligodendrocytes
(C) microglial cells
(D) both A & B

45. Motor nerve fibres begin to develop -
(A) during 4th week
(B) during 5th week
(C) during 6th week
(D) during 8th week

46. Derivatives of neural crest are all except-
(A) odontoblasts
(B) dentine
(C) cementoblasts
(D) dental papilla

47. Derivatives of neural crest are all except-
(A) piamater
(B) arachnoidmater
(C) duramater
(D) melanoblast

48. Derivatives of neural crest are all except-
(A) 5th cranial nerve sensory ganglia
(B) 7th cranial nerve sensory ganglia
(C) 3rd cranial nerve sensory ganglia
(D) 10th cranial nerve sensory ganglia

49. Derivatives of neural crest are all except-
(A) Ciliary ganglion
(B) otic ganglion
(C) geniculate ganglion
(D) submandibular ganglion

50. Derivatives of neural crest are all except-
(A) adrenal medulla
(B) Schwann cells
(C) adrenal cortex
(D) C cells of thyroid

51. Myelination of neurons starts at the age of-
(A) 4th week
(B) 40th day
(C) 4th month
(D) 14th week

52. Length of spinal cord is equal to vertebral column at the age of-
(A) third week
(B) thirtieth week
(C) third month of intrauterine life
(D) sixth month of intrauterine life

53. At birth level of spinal cord is-
(A) equal to vertebral column
(B) L3 level
(C) L5 level
(D) L1 level

54. In adults level of spinal cord is-
(A) equal to vertebral column
(B) L3 level
(C) L5 level
(D) L1 level

55. Widest part of spinal cord is-
(A) cervical
(B) thoracic
(C) lumbar
(D) sacral

56. Thinnest part of spinal cord is-
(A) cervical
(B) thoracic
(C) lumbar
(D) sacral

57. Factors responsible for neural tube defects are-
(A) hyperthermia
(B) valproic acid
(C) hypervitaminosis A
(D) All of the above

58. Basal plate of medulla oblongata have somatic efferent nuclei in-
(A) medial group
(B) intermediate group
(C) lateral group
(D) none of the above

59. Basal plate of medulla oblongata have special efferent nuclei in-
(A) medial group
(B) intermediate group
(C) lateral group
(D) none of the above

60. Basal plate of medulla oblongata have general visceral efferent nuclei in-
(A) medial group
(B) intermediate group
(C) lateral group
(D) none of the above

61. Olivary nuclei develops from-
(A) rhombic lip
(B) bulbopontine extension
(C) somatic efferent column
(D) somatic afferent column

62. Gracile & cuneate nuclei develops from -
(A) rhombic lip
(B) bulbopontine extension
(C) somatic efferent column
(D) somatic afferent column

63. Pontine nuclei develops from-
(A) rhombic lip
(B) bulbopontine extension
(C) somatic efferent column
(D) somatic afferent column

64. Vermis of the cerebellum can be seen earliest at -
(A) eighth week
(B) tenth week
(C) twelfth week
(D) fourteenth week

65. Morphologically most primitive part of brain vesicle is-
(A) hind brain
(B) midbrain
(C) forebrain
(D) none of the above

66. Structures derived from alar lamina of mid brain are –
(A) colliculi
(B) red nucleus
(C) substantia nigra
(D) all of the above

67. Structures derived from basal lamina of mid brain are –
(A) occulomotor nucleus
(B) trochlear nucleus
(C) Edinger Westphal nucleus
(D) all of the above

68. Commissural fibres appearing earliest are-
(A) corpus callosum
(B) anterior commissure
(C) posterior commissure
(D) lamina terminalis

69. Commissural fibres appearing second are-
(A) corpus callosum
(B) hippocampal commissure
(C) anterior commissure
(D) lamina terminalis

70. Corpus callosum appears at the age of–
(A) sixth week
(B) seventh week
(C) eighth week
(D) tenth week

71. All cranial nerve nuclei appears at the age of-
(A) third week
(B) fourth week
(C) sixth week
(D) eighth week

72. Cerebellum starts forming at the age of-
(A) tenth week
(B) fourth week
(C) sixth week
(D) eighth week

73. Pineal body appears at the age of –
(A) sixth week
(B) seventh week
(C) eighth week
(D) tenth week

74. Rathke's pouch appears at the age of-
(A) third week
(B) fourth week
(C) sixth week
(D) eighth week

75. Cerebral hemispheres appears at the age of-
(A) third week
(B) fourth week
(C) fifth week
(D) sixth week

76. Cerebral cortex and Purkinje's cells appears at the age of-
(A) tenth week
(B) eleventh week
(C) twelfth week
(D) fourteenth week

77. Dentate nucleus of cerebellum is seen at –
(A) eleventh week
(B) twelfth week
(C) fourteenth week
(D) fifteenth week

Answer Sheet

1 (C)	2 (C)	3 (D)	4 (C)	5 (A)	6 (C)	7 (B)	8 (D)	9 (C)	10 (A)
11 (B)	12 (C)	13 (D)	14 (A)	15 (B)	16 (A)	17 (C)	18 (D)	19 (B)	20 (A)
21 (D)	22 (B)	23 (B)	24 (D)	25 (A)	26 (C)	27 (B)	28 (C)	29 (A)	30 (A)
31 (B)	32 (D)	33 (B)	34 (A)	35 (B)	36 (A)	37 (C)	38 (C)	39 (A)	40 (A)
41 (C)	42 (B)	43 (A)	44 (B)	45 (A)	46 (C)	47 (C)	48 (C)	49 (C)	50 (C)
51 (C)	52 (C)	53 (B)	54 (D)	55 (A)	56 (B)	57 (D)	58 (A)	59 (B)	60 (C)
61 (B)	62 (D)	63 (B)	64 (C)	65 (B)	66 (D)	67 (D)	68 (B)	69 (B)	70 (D)
71 (B)	72 (D)	73 (B)	74 (A)	75 (C)	76 (C)	77 (D)			

EXPLANATIONS

1 **(C) The anterior and posterior neuropores of developing neural tube close during 4th week of development.**

2 **(C)** Third ventricle is the cavity of diencephalon and lies between two thalami and hypothalamus. In communicates dorsally with aqueduct of midbrain and on other side with lateral ventricles through foramina of Monroe.

3 **(D)** The structure developing from diencephalon is Neurohypophysis that form part, of pituitary gland Adenohypophysis develops from an ectodermal Rathke's pouch.

4 **(C)** The tip of conus medullaris end at level L3 at birth. In adult it ends at level L1.

5 **(A)** The general somatic efferent column of basal lamina is represented in pons by abducent nucleus.

6 **(C)** Nucleus ambiguous represents special visceral efferent column in medulla oblongata.

7 **(B)** Hippocampus is derived from telencephalon. The pineal gland hypothalamus and optic nerve are all derived from diencephalon.

8 **(D)** The pontine flexure develops between metencephalon (pons) and the mylencephalon (medulla oblongata). The pontine flexure results in lateral expansion of walls of metencephalon and mylencephalon stretching the roof of fourth ventricle and widening the floor of IVth ventricle (rhomboid fossa).

9 **(B)** The sulcus limitans separates the alar and basal lamina. It is found in developing spinal cord and on the surface of rhomboid fossa.

10 **(A)** The spina bifida with meningo-myelocele describes the herniation of spinal cord through a defect in vertebrae along with its meninges.

11 **(B)** The cerebellum develops from rhombic lip of alar lamina. The rhombic lips of two sides fuse in midline to form the vermis part of cerebellum.

12 **(C)** The choroid plexus of forth ventricle is derived from roof plate of hind brain. The alar plate give rise to sensory neurons and basal plates gives rise to interneurons.

13 **(D)** Myelinated pre-ganglionic sympathetic neurons have their cell bodies in intermediate lateral cells column of spinal cord.

14 **(A)** The piamater is derived from the neural crest cells as part of pia-arachnoid.

Chapter 10

Endocrine Glands

1. Thyroid glands develop from-
(A) 2nd pharyngeal pouch
(B) 3rd pharyngeal pouch
(C) 4th pharyngeal pouch
(D) Thyroglossal duct from floor of primitive pharynx

2. Adenohypophysis develops from-
(A) Neural diverticulum
(B) Midbrain
(C) Hindbrain
(D) Rathke's pouch from roof of stomodaeum

3. The Supra-renal cortex develops from-
(A) Coelomic epithelium
(B) Neural crest
(C) Surface ectoderm
(D) Midgut

4. The Supra-renal medulla develops from-
(A) Neuroectoderm
(B) Neural crest
(C) Mesoderm
(D) Endoderm

5. The pineal gland develops from-
(A) Telencephalon
(B) Metencephalon
(C) Roof plate of diencephalon
(D) Myelencephalon

6. The Superior parathyroid develops from-
(A) 4th pharyngeal pouch
(B) 3rd pharyngeal pouch
(C) 2nd pharyngeal pouch
(D) 1st pharyngeal pouch

7. The inferior parathyroid develops from-
(A) 4th pharyngeal pouch
(B) 3rd pharyngeal pouch
(C) 2nd pharyngeal pouch
(D) 1st pharyngeal pouch

8. Infundibular diverticulum develops in the floor of third ventricle at the age of–
(A) third week
(B) fourth week
(C) fifth week
(D) eighth week

9. Rathke's pouch projects from the roof of stomodaeum at the age of –
(A) third week
(B) fourth week
(C) fifth week
(D) eighth week

10. Suprarenal gland begins to develop at the age of –
(A) third week
(B) fourth week
(C) fifth week
(D) eighth week

11. Rathke's pouch loses its connection with the oral cavity at the age of –
(A) third week
(B) fourth week
(C) fifth week
(D) eighth week

12. Craniopharyngiomas are the tumors arising from –
(A) pineal gland
(B) pituitary gland
(C) remnants of Rathke's pouch
(D) all of the above

13. Anterior part of pituitary is derived from –
(A) endoderm
(B) mesoderm
(C) ectoderm
(D) all of the above

14. Cells of the pineal glands are –
(A) neuroglial cells
(B) part of diencephalon
(C) both are true
(D) none of the above

15. Suprarenal gland develops from –
(A) endoderm & ectoderm
(B) mesoderm & ectoderm
(C) mesoderm & endoderm
(D) endoderm, ectoderm & mesoderm

16. Cells of foetal cortex are seen in which zone of definitive cortex of suprarenal gland –
(A) zona glomerulosa
(B) zona fasciculata
(C) zona reticulosa
(D) all of the above

17. Which zone is seen in the adrenal gland at the time of birth –
(A) zona glomerulosa
(B) zona fasciculata
(C) zona reticulosa
(D) both A & B

18. Zona reticulosa is recognisable at the age of-
(A) first year of life
(B) second year of life
(C) third year of life
(D) fifth year of life

19. Thymus gland develops from –
(A) second pouch
(B) third pouch
(C) fourth pouch
(D) fifth pouch

20. Superior parathyroid gland develops from –
(A) second pouch
(B) third pouch
(C) fourth pouch
(D) fifth pouch

21. Inferior parathyroid gland develops from –
(A) second pouch
(B) third pouch
(C) fourth pouch
(D) fifth pouch

22. Fourth pouch contributes to-
(A) superior parathyroid & thymus
(B) superior parathyroid & thyroid
(C) inferior parathyroid & thymus
(D) inferior parathyroid & thyroid

23. Third pouch contributes to-
(A) superior parathyroid & thymus
(B) superior parathyroid & thyroid
(C) inferior parathyroid & thymus
(D) inferior parathyroid & thyroid

24. Parafollicular C cells of thyroid are derived from-
(A) second pouch
(B) third pouch
(C) fourth pouch
(D) ultimobranchial body

25. Parathyroid glands develop from-
(A) second pouch & third pouch
(B) third pouch & fourth pouch
(C) fourth pouch
(D) ultimobranchial body

26. Ectopic thyroid tissue is seen in –
(A) pons
(B) cerebellum
(C) cerebrum
(D) corpus callosum

27. Ectopic thyroid tissue is seen in-
(A) larynx
(B) trachea
(C) oesophagus
(D) all of the above

28. Thyroid gland reach its definitive position by-
(A) fifth week
(B) sixth week
(C) seventh week
(D) eighth week

29. Thyroid gland formation starts by-
(A) fifth week
(B) sixth week
(C) seventh week
(D) eighth week

30. Pancreatic bud appears at the age of –
(A) third week
(B) fourth week
(C) fifth week
(D) sixth week

31. Pancreatic islets appears at the age of–
(A) third week
(B) fourth week
(C) third month
(D) fourth month

32. Insulin secretion from pancreatic islets appears at the age of –
(A) third month
(B) fourth month
(C) fifth month
(D) sixth month

Answer Sheet

1 (D)	2 (D)	3 (A)	4 (B)	5 (C)	6 (A)	7 (B)	8 (A)	9 (B)	10 (C)
11 (D)	12 (C)	13 (C)	14 (C)	15 (B)	16 (C)	17 (D)	18 (C)	19 (B)	20 (C)
21 (B)	22 (B)	23 (C)	24 (D)	25 (B)	26 (A)	27 (D)	28 (C)	29 (A)	30 (A)
31 (C)	32 (C)								

EXPLANATIONS

1 **(D)** Thyroid gland develops from thyroglossal duct, arise from the endoderm of floor of primitive pharynx. The site of duct marked in adult tongue as foramen caecum.

2 **(D)** Adenohypophysis develops from Rathke's pouch that is an ectodermal diverticulum growing from roof of primitive mouth or stomodeum. Remnants of Rathke's pouch may give rise to Craniopharyngiomas.

3 **(A)** Supra-renal cortex develops from coelomic epithelium. The first wave of proliferation of coelomic epithelium give rise to foetal cortex that is surrounded by adult cortex. The foetal cortex after birth undergoes regression.

4 **(B)** The supra-renal medulla develops from neural crest as chromaffin tissue that stain yellow-brown with chromium salts. The chromaffin cells are also found near abdominal aorta, but most of them disappear after birth.

5 **(C)** The pineal gland develops from caudal end of roof plate of diencephalon. It is a derivative of alar lamina.

6 **(A)** The superior parathyroid develops from fourth pharyngeal pouch. The inferior parathyroid develops from third pharyngeal pouch, that also give rise to thymus gland. The thymus gland pulls inferior parathyroid to a lower level that superior parathyroid.

Section - 4

Histology

Chapter 1

Epithelial Tissue

1. One micrometre is equal to-
(A) 0.001 mm
(B) 0.001 mtrs
(C) 10-9 mtr
(D) 10-10 mtr

2. While processing the tissue for paraffin embedding, dehydration is done by immersing the tissue in -
(A) Alcohol only
(B) Xylol only
(C) Mixture of alcohol and xylol
(D) Formalin

3. Haematoxylin is a basic dye and it stains-
(A) The basic components of a cell only
(B) The acidic components of a cell only
(C) Both basic and acidic components of a cell
(D) None of these

4. The optical parts of a light microscope involved in magnification is the-
(A) condenser and filter
(B) eyepiece only
(C) objective only
(D) both objective and eyepiece

5. 9 + 2 pattern of microtubules is present in -
(A) Glycocalyx
(B) Microvilli
(C) Stereocilia
(D) Cilia

6. Transitional epithelium is found in-
(A) Uterus
(B) Urinary bladder
(C) Gall bladder
(D) Vagina

7. In pseudostratified columnar epithelium-
(A) all cells are attached to the basement membrane
(B) all cell do not reach the surface
(C) all nuclei are situated at different levels
(D) all of the are correct

8. Stomach is lined by -
(A) simple columnar epithelium
(B) stratified squamous epithelium
(C) pseudostratified columnar epithelium
(D) simple cuboidal epithelium

9. Glycocalyx present in the absorptive epithelium of small intestine-
(A) increase the surface area for absorption
(B) transports the absorbed material
(C) concentrates ions prior to absorption
(D) participates in the digestion of carbohydrates

10. Columnar epithelium has –
(A) flat nucleus
(B) round nucleus
(C) oval nucleus
(D) all of the above

11. Cuboidal epithelium has –
(A) flat nucleus
(B) round nucleus
(C) oval nucleus
(D) all of the above

12. Squamous epithelium has –
(A) flat nucleus
(B) round nucleus
(C) oval nucleus
(D) all of the above

13. True about zona occludens or tight junctions is all except-
(A) located near basal part of cell
(B) seen in epithelium of urinary bladder
(C) located near apical part of cell
(D) prevents passage of material

14. Ion responsible for cellular cohesion is-
(A) magnesium
(B) potassium
(C) calcium
(D) all of the above

15. Cuboidal epithelium is seen in all except -
(A) thyroid follicle
(B) palpebral conjunctiva
(C) surface of ovary
(D) PCT of kidneys

16. Simple squamous epithelium is seen in all except -
(A) mesothelium
(B) surface epithelium of ovary
(C) alveoli of lungs
(D) bowman's capsule of kidneys

17. Simple columnar epithelium is seen in-
(A) stomach
(B) gall bladder
(C) intestine
(D) all of the above

18. Columnar ciliated epithelium is seen in-
(A) stomach
(B) gall bladder
(C) uterine tube
(D) all of the above

19. Pseudostratified columnar epithelium is seen in -
(A) nasal cavity
(B) trachea
(C) bronchi
(D) all of the above

20. Pseudostratified columnar epithelium with Stereocilia is seen in -
(A) epididymis
(B) vas deferens
(C) nasal cavity
(D) A & B

21. Stratified cuboidal epithelium is seen in -
(A) sweat gland
(B) gall bladder
(C) palpebral conjunctiva
(D) all of the above

22. Stratified columnar epithelium is seen in -
(A) stomach
(B) gall bladder
(C) intestine
(D) palpebral conjunctiva

23. Stratified squamous epithelium has –
(A) squamous cells
(B) polyhedral cells
(C) columnar cells
(D) all of the above

24. Epithelium of cardiovascular system develops from-
(A) endoderm
(B) mesoderm
(C) ectoderm
(D) all of the above

25. Epithelium of gastrointestinal system develops from-
(A) endoderm
(B) mesoderm
(C) ectoderm
(D) all of the above

26. Epithelium of integumentary system develops from-
(A) endoderm
(B) mesoderm
(C) ectoderm
(D) all of the above

27. Large umbrella cells are seen in-
(A) stratified squamous epithelium
(B) stratified columnar epithelium
(C) transitional epithelium
(D) all of the above

28. Flagellum is seen in-
(A) sperm
(B) respiratory epithelium
(C) intestinal epithelium
(D) epididymis

29. Cilia is seen in-
(A) sperm
(B) respiratory epithelium
(C) intestinal epithelium
(D) epididymis

30. Stereocilia is seen in-
(A) sperm
(B) respiratory epithelium
(C) intestinal epithelium
(D) epididymis

31. Microvilli is seen in-
(A) sperm
(B) respiratory epithelium
(C) intestinal epithelium
(D) epididymis

32. Brush border is seen in-
(A) proximal convoluted tubule
(B) respiratory epithelium
(C) intestinal epithelium
(D) epididymis

33. Simple squamous epithelium is seen in all except-
(A) proximal convoluted tubule
(B) internal ear
(C) serous pericardium
(D) alveoli of lung

34. Simple cuboidal epithelium is seen in all except-
(A) ducts of pancreas
(B) choroid plexus
(C) thyroid follicles
(D) surface covering of ovary

35. Simple cuboidal epithelium is seen in -
(A) pigment cell layer of retina
(B) choroid plexus
(C) inner surface of lens
(D) all of the above

36. Simple columnar epithelium is seen in-
(A) stomach
(B) large intestine
(C) gall bladder
(D) all of the above

37. Ciliated columnar epithelium is seen in all except -
(A) respiratory tract
(B) uterus
(C) uterine tube
(D) roof of the nose

38. Columnar epithelium with striated border is seen in -
(A) proximal convoluted tubule of kidney
(B) stomach
(C) gall bladder
(D) surface covering of ovary

39. Non ciliated pseudostratified columnar epithelium is seen in -
(A) auditory tube
(B) ductus deferens
(C) male urethra membranous part
(D) all of the above

40. Ciliated pseudostratified columnar epithelium is seen in -
(A) trachea
(B) large bronchi
(C) epididymis
(D) all of the above

41. Pseudostratified columnar epithelium with Stereocilia is seen in -
(A) epididymis
(B) ductus deferens
(C) male urethra membranous part
(D) all of the above

42. Stratified squamous epithelium is seen in –
(A) cornea
(B) vagina
(C) tongue
(D) all of the above

43. Transitional epithelium is seen in all except -
(A) ureter
(B) penile urethra
(C) urinary bladder
(D) renal pelvis

44. Stratified low columnar epithelium is seen in all except-
(A) ducts of salivary glands
(B) ducts of sweat gland
(C) ovi-duct
(D) pancreatic duct

Answer Sheet

1 (A)	2 (A)	3 (B)	4 (D)	5 (D)	6 (B)	7 (D)	8 (A)	9 (C)	10 (C)
11 (B)	12 (A)	13 (A)	14 (C)	15 (B)	16 (B)	17 (D)	18 (C)	19 (D)	20 (D)
21 (A)	22 (D)	23 (D)	24 (B)	25 (A)	26 (C)	27 (C)	28 (A)	29 (B)	30 (D)
31 (C)	32 (A)	33 (A)	34 (A)	35 (D)	36 (D)	37 (D)	38 (C)	39 (D)	40 (D)
41 (A)	42 (D)	43 (B)	44 (C)						

Chapter 2

Connective Tissue

1. Plasma cells are derived from-
(A) monocytes
(B) basophils
(C) T lymphocyte
(D) B lymphpcytes

2. Connective tissue is made up of-
(A) cells
(B) fibres
(C) ground substance
(D) all of the above

3. Which of the following is not true about fixed macrophage? It-
(A) contains many lysosomes
(B) has basophilic cytoplasm
(C) can be stained with vital dyes
(D) is involved in phagocytosis

4. Large number of elastic fibres are present in-
(A) tendon
(B) ligamentum nuchae
(C) basement membrane
(D) aponeurosis

5. Which of the following is not true about collagen? it-
(A) constitutes 30% of the dry body weight
(B) is synthesised by fibroblasts
(C) gives gelatin on denaturation
(D) is composed of mucopolysaccharides

6. Mucoid tissue is seen in –
(A) panniculus adiposus
(B) Wharton's jelly
(C) reticular tissue
(D) elastic tissue

7. Regular dense connective tissue is seen in all except-
(A) tendon
(B) ligaments
(C) skin
(D) aponeurosis

8. Fixed cells in the connective tissue are-
(A) fibroblast
(B) mesenchymal cells
(C) histiocytes
(D) all of the above

9. Fixed cells in the connective tissue are-
(A) fibrocytes
(B) fixed macrophages
(C) adipocytes
(D) all of the above

10. Wandering cells in the connective tissue are all except -
(A) plasma cells
(B) mast cells
(C) fixed macrophages
(D) leucocytes

11. Most common cells in connective tissue is-
(A) fibroblast
(B) mesenchymal cells
(C) histiocytes
(D) all of the above

12. True about fibroblast is-
(A) flat, fusiform in shape and slender processes
(B) secrets fibres and ground substances
(C) euchromatic nucleus with prominent nucleoli
(D) all of the above

13. True about fibroblast is-
(A) associated with collagen fibres
(B) old inactive and mature cells are called fibrocytes
(C) in wound healing become contractile myofibroblasts
(D) all of the above

14. True about undifferentiated mesenchymal cells is-
(A) stellate in shape and slender processes
(B) are pluripotent and may be converted to other cells on stimulation
(C) resemble fibroblasts and are called adventitial cells
(D) all of the above

15. True about adipocyte is-
(A) called signet ring
(B) incapable of division
(C) supported by reticular fibres
(D) all of the above

16. True about histiocytes is all except -
(A) flat, fusiform in shape and slender processes
(B) irregular in shape with filopodia
(C) eccentrically placed indented nucleus
(D) derived from monocytes

17. True about macrophage is-
(A) phagocytic function
(B) activates B lymphocytes
(C) forms multinucleated giant cell on stimulation
(D) all of the above

18. True about plasma cell is all except -
(A) oval cell with basophilic cytoplasm
(B) cart wheel nucleus
(C) derived from monocytes
(D) derived from B lymphocytes

19. Russell's bodies are seen in-
(A) mast cells
(B) monocytes
(C) plasma cells
(D) all of the above

20. Type I collagen is found in all except-
(A) bones
(B) tendons
(C) cartilage
(D) dermis

21. Type II collagen is found in -
(A) bones
(B) basement membrane
(C) cartilage
(D) blood vessels

22. Type III collagen is found in -
(A) reticular fibres
(B) basement membrane
(C) cartilage
(D) blood vessels

23. Type IV collagen is found in -
(A) bones
(B) basement membrane
(C) cartilage
(D) blood vessels

24. Type V collagen is found in -
(A) bones
(B) basement membrane
(C) cartilage
(D) blood vessels

25. Type V collagen is found in -
(A) bones
(B) basement membrane
(C) foetal membranes
(D) dermis

26. Collagen fibres are stained red by-
(A) Van Gieson method
(B) Masson's trichome
(C) silver impregnation
(D) all of the above

27. Collagen fibres are stained by-
(A) Van Gieson method
(B) Masson's trichome
(C) silver impregnation
(D) all of the above

28. Collagen fibres are stained blue by-
(A) Van Gieson method
(B) Masson's trichome
(C) silver impregnation
(D) all of the above

29. Collagen fibres are stained brown by-
(A) Van Gieson method
(B) Masson's trichome
(C) silver impregnation
(D) all of the above

30. Reticular fibres are stained black by-
(A) Van Gieson method
(B) Masson's trichome
(C) silver impregnation
(D) all of the above

31. True about adult type/yellow type of adipose tissue is all except-
(A) single – unilocular cells
(B) flat peripheral nucleus
(C) many mitochondria
(D) few mitochondria

32. True about embryonic type/brown type of adipose tissue is all except-
(A) large – multilocular cells
(B) spherical central nucleus
(C) many mitochondria
(D) few mitochondria

33. True about reticular fibres is-
(A) collagen type III fibres
(B) supportive framework in lymphoid organs
(C) stained with silver salts – argyrophilic
(D) all of the above

34. All are structural glycoproteins of connective tissue except –
(A) laminin
(B) glycosaminoglycan
(C) chondronectin
(D) fibronectin

35. Glycoproteins of the dermal connective tissue is –
(A) laminin
(B) glycosaminoglycan
(C) chondronectin
(D) fibronectin

36. Structural glycoproteins found in the basement membrane is –
(A) laminin
(B) glycosaminoglycan
(C) chondronectin
(D) fibronectin

37. Elastic fibres are found in –
(A) large arteries
(B) ligamentum flava
(C) ligamentum nuchae
(D) all of the above

38. Collagen fibres are synthesised by –
(A) fibroblasts & myoblasts
(B) chondroblasts & osteoblasts
(C) odontoblasts
(D) all of the above

39. Connective tissue basophil is name given to-
(A) leucocytes
(B) mast cells
(C) plasma cells
(D) adipocyte

40. Collagen fibres are made up of –
(A) double helix
(B) triple helix
(C) single chain
(D) none of the above

41. Procollagen chain is made up of-
(A) glycine
(B) hydroxylysine
(C) hydroxyproline
(D) all of the above

42. Fibres seen in lens capsule of the eye are-
(A) type I
(B) type II
(C) type III
(D) type IV

43. Fibres seen in vitreous body of the eye are-
(A) type I
(B) type II
(C) type III
(D) type IV

44. Elastic fibres are specifically stained with-
(A) orcein
(B) aldehyde fuschin
(C) verhoeff's method
(D) all of the above

45. Fibroblasts produce –
(A) collagen fibres
(B) elastic fibres
(C) reticular fibres
(D) all of the above

46. Filopodia or irregular microvilli are seen in-
(A) fibroblasts
(B) adipocytes
(C) mast cells
(D) lymphocytes

47. Mast cells are stained with –
(A) PAS
(B) toluidine blue
(C) alcian blue
(D) all of the above

48. Components of human fat cells are –
(A) oleic acid
(B) linoleic acid
(C) palmitic acid
(D) all of the above

Answer Sheet

1 (D)	2 (D)	3 (B)	4 (B)	5 (D)	6 (B)	7 (C)	8 (D)	9 (D)	10 (C)
11 (A)	12 (D)	13 (D)	14 (D)	15 (D)	16 (A)	17 (D)	18 (C)	19 (C)	20 (C)
21 (C)	22 (A)	23 (B)	24 (D)	25 (C)	26 (A)	27 (D)	28 (B)	29 (C)	30 (C)
31 (C)	32 (D)	33 (D)	34 (B)	35 (D)	36 (A)	37 (D)	38 (D)	39 (B)	40 (B)
41 (D)	42 (D)	43 (B)	44 (D)	45 (D)	46 (C)	47 (D)	48 (D)		

Chapter **3**

Cartilage & Bone

1. A section of hyaline cartilage can be identified by the presence of-
(A) Homogeneous matrix
(B) Elastic fibres
(C) Collagen fibres
(D) Chondrocytes arranged in row

2. Elastic cartilage is present in-
(A) Tracheal ring
(B) Epiglottis
(C) Intervertebral disc
(D) Costal cartilage

3. Growth of cartilage depends on-
(A) growth hormone
(B) somatomedin C
(C) vascularity of tissue
(D) all of the above

4. True about cartilage is-
(A) avascular structure
(B) no nerves are present
(C) regeneration is poor
(D) all of the above

5. Perichondrium is absent in-
(A) Elastic cartilage and hyaline cartilage
(B) Hyaline cartilage and cellular cartilage
(C) Fibrocartilage and articular cartilage
(D) Costal cartilage and ear pinna

6. True about the nourishment of the cartilage is-
(A) highly vascular & aerobic
(B) diffusion & aerobic
(C) diffusion & anaerobic
(D) none of the above

7. Which of the following feature is not true about cartilage?
(A) Firm and flexible
(B) highly vascular
(C) Insensitive
(D) Poor in regeneration

8. Chondrocytes are-
(A) Derived from monocyte
(B) Involved in phagocytosis
(C) Polyhedral in shape
(D) Found in lacunae

9. Alkaline phosphatases is secreted by-
(A) chondroblast
(B) chondrocytes
(C) chondroblasts & chondrocytes both
(D) none of the above

10. Hyaline cartilage is seen in-
(A) cricoid cartilage
(B) costal cartilage
(C) epiphyseal cartilage
(D) all of the above

11. Elastic cartilage is seen in all except-
(A) corniculate cartilage
(B) cuneiform cartilage
(C) cricoid cartilage
(D) epiglottis

12. Cartilage responsible for the growth of long bone is-
(A) articular cartilage
(B) fibrocartilage
(C) hyaline cartilage
(D) elastic cartilage

13. Typical features of hyaline cartilage is-
(A) homogenous basophilic matrix
(B) cell nests
(C) perichondrium covering
(D) all of the above

14. Typical features of articular cartilage are all except-
(A) homogeneous basophilic matrix
(B) cell nests
(C) perichondrium present
(D) perichondrium absent

15. Typical features of fibrocartilage are all except -
(A) dense bundles of collagen
(B) cell nests
(C) perichondrium absent
(D) rows of chondrocytes

16. Typical features of elastic cartilage are-
(A) nonhomogeneous matrix
(B) cell nests
(C) perichondrium covering present
(D) chondrocytes with eccentric nuclei

17. Elliptical young chondrocytes are seen in-
(A) cell nests
(B) just beneath the perichondrium
(C) rows of chondrocytes
(D) free in homogenous matrix

18. Eccentrically placed nuclei in chondrocytes are seen in-
(A) hyaline cartilage
(B) elastic cartilage
(C) fibrocartilage
(D) all of the above

19. Defects in cartilage are generally filled by-
(A) fibrocartilage
(B) fibrous tissue
(C) no ability to heal
(D) bone formation

20. Collagen fibres in cartilage are –
(A) type I
(B) type II
(C) type III
(D) type IV

21. Collagen fibres in Fibrocartilage are –
(A) type I
(B) type II
(C) type III
(D) type IV

22. Cartilage which may calcify with age is-
(A) hyaline cartilage
(B) elastic cartilage
(C) fibrocartilage
(D) all of the above

23. Periosteum is absent over the following except-
(A) Articular surface of bone
(B) Sesamoid bone
(C) Site of attachment of tendons and ligaments to the bone
(D) Outer table of flat bone

24. Osteocytes can be identified by the presence of -
(A) Many nuclei
(B) Lacuna around the cell
(C) lysosomes
(D) ingested particles

25. Alkaline phosphatase activity can be demonstrated in-
(A) osteoblast
(B) osteocytes
(C) osteoclast
(D) osteoprogenitor cells

26. Spongy bone can be identified histologically by the presence of-
(A) Haversian canal
(B) Bony trabeculae and marrow cavity
(C) Interstitial lamellae
(D) Volkmann's canal

27. The vitamin necessary for absorption of calcium from small intestine is-
(A) Vitamin A
(B) Vitamin C
(C) Vitamin D
(D) Vitamin E

28. Compact bone is seen in-
(A) shaft of long bones
(B) tables of flat bones
(C) shell of short bones
(D) all of the above

29. Cancellous or spongy bone is seen in-
(A) end of long bones
(B) diploe of flat bones
(C) short bones
(D) all of the above

30. Periosteum is not seen on-
(A) pisiform
(B) tibia
(C) talus
(D) ulna

31. Periosteum is not seen at-
(A) sesamoid bones
(B) articular ends of long bone
(C) tendon & ligament attachment areas
(D) all of the above

32. Sharpey's fibres are seen in-
(A) cartilage
(B) bone
(C) mylinated nerves
(D) none of the above

33. Collagen fibres present in bones are-
(A) type I
(B) type II
(C) type III
(D) all of the above

34. Most abundant component of the bone is-
(A) cells
(B) inorganic salts of calcium
(C) type I collagen fibres
(D) ground substance

35. Osteoprogenitor cell which is mesenchymal in origin give rise to-
(A) osteocytes
(B) osteoblasts
(C) osteoclasts
(D) all of the above

36. Shape of the osteoblast is –
(A) oval with cytoplasmic processes
(B) cuboidal
(C) large irregular giant cell
(D) none of the above

37. Shape of the osteoclast is –
(A) oval with cytoplasmic processes
(B) cuboidal
(C) large irregular giant cell
(D) none of the above

38. All is true about osteoblast except-
(A) cuboidal in shape
(B) basophilic cytoplasm
(C) alkaline phosphatases positive
(D) acid phosphatases positive

39. All is true about osteoclast except-
(A) multinucleated giant shaped
(B) derived from blood monocytes
(C) alkaline phosphatases positive
(D) acid phosphatases positive

40. Cell present in Howship's lacuna is-
(A) osteoblasts
(B) osteocytes
(C) osteoclasts
(D) all of the above

41. Bone cell derived from blood cell is-
(A) osteoblasts
(B) osteocytes
(C) osteoclasts
(D) all of the above

42. True about Haversian canal of bone is-
(A) lie along parallel axis of long bone
(B) lined with endosteum
(C) having osteoprogenitor cells
(D) all of the above

43. Essential vitamins for bone formation are all except–
(A) vit A
(B) vit D
(C) vit E
(D) vit C

44. Vitamin necessary for ossification is-
(A) vit A
(B) vit D
(C) vit E
(D) vit C

45. Vitamin necessary for calcium absorption from GIT –
(A) vit A
(B) vit D
(C) vit E
(D) vit C

46. Hormones playing important role in bone growth are-
(A) growth hormone
(B) calcitonin
(C) parathyroid hormone
(D) all of the above

47. Boundary between each Haversian system is called as-
(A) Haversian line
(B) interstitial line
(C) cement line
(D) lamellar line

48. Bone lining cells are -
(A) flattened cells and can convert into osteoblasts in need
(B) seen on endosteal surface
(C) seen on periosteal surface
(D) all of the above

49. Fusion of epiphysis and diaphysis in growing bone is-
(A) symphysis
(B) synostosis
(C) syndesmosis
(D) none of the above

50. Bone eating cells are-
(A) osteoclasts
(B) osteoblasts
(C) osteocytes
(D) osteoprogenitor cells

Answer Sheet

1 (A)	2 (B)	3 (D)	4 (D)	5 (C)	6 (C)	7 (B)	8 (D)	9 (B)	10 (D)
11 (C)	12 (C)	13 (D)	14 (C)	15 (B)	16 (B)	17 (B)	18 (B)	19 (B)	20 (B)
21 (A)	22 (A)	23 (D)	24 (B)	25 (A)	26 (B)	27 (C)	28 (D)	29 (D)	30 (A)
31 (D)	32 (B)	33 (A)	34 (C)	35 (B)	36 (B)	37 (C)	38 (D)	39 (C)	40 (C)
41 (C)	42 (D)	43 (C)	44 (B)	45 (B)	46 (D)	47 (C)	48 (D)	49 (B)	50 (A)

Chapter 4

Lymphoid Tissue

1. Thymus has the following features except that it-
   (A) Is a central lymphoid organ
   (B) Has no reticular fibres and reticular cells
   (C) Involutes after puberty
   (D) Is formed by B lymphocytes

2. Thymus- dependent zone of a lymph node is-
   (A) cortex
   (B) paracortex
   (C) medullary cord
   (D) medullary sinuses

3. First line of defence is provided by-
   (A) neutrophils & macrophages
   (B) surface epithelium
   (C) specific immune response evoked by lymphocytes
   (D) none of the above

4. Second line of defence is provided by-
   (A) neutrophils & macrophages
   (B) surface epithelium
   (C) specific immune response evoked by lymphocytes
   (D) none of the above

5. Third line of defence is provided by-
   (A) neutrophils & macrophages
   (B) surface epithelium
   (C) specific immune response evoked by lymphocytes
   (D) none of the above

6. The main type of Immunoglobin present in various glandular secretion is-
   (A) IgG
   (B) IgA
   (C) IgM
   (D) IgE

7. Immunoglobulins are secreted by-
   (A) B lymphocytes
   (B) plasma cells
   (C) T lymphocytes
   (D) mast cells

8. Most common Immunoglobin is-
   (A) IgG
   (B) IgM
   (C) IgA
   (D) IgD

9. Immunoglobulins crossing the placenta is-
(A) IgG
(B) IgM
(C) IgA
(D) IgD

10. The percentage of T lymphocytes present in blood is-
(A) 80
(B) 40
(C) 20
(D) 10

11. Which of the following is not an antigen-presenting cell?
(A) Langerhans's cell
(B) follicular dendritic cell
(C) M cell
(D) Mast cell

12. Which of the following is an antigen-presenting cell?
(A) Langerhans's cell
(B) follicular dendritic cell in lymphoid organ
(C) M cell
(D) All of the above

13. White pulp of spleen can be identified differentially from the lymphatic nodule of lymph node by the presence of
(A) Germinal centre
(B) Cornea
(C) Central arteriole
(D) Lymphocytes

14. Crypts of palatine tonsil are lined by
(A) Simple squamous epithelium
(B) Stratified squamous nonkeratinised epithelium
(C) Pseudo stratified columnar epithelium
(D) Stratified squamous keratinised epithelium

15. True about IgA is-
(A) present in body secretions
(B) about 15% of total immunoglobulins
(C) protects mucosal membranes
(D) all of the above

16. In colostrum the immunoglobulin present is-
(A) IgG
(B) IgA
(C) IgM
(D) all of the above

17. Surface of mast cells presents-
(A) IgG
(B) IgE
(C) IgM
(D) IgA

18. Hassall's corpuscles are present in-
(A) Lymph node
(B) Spleen
(C) Thymus
(D) Tonsil

19. A section of lymph nodes can be identified by the presence of-
(A) Thick trabeculae
(B) Interlobular septum
(C) White pulp
(D) Subcapsular sinus

20. Splenic sinuses are lined by-
(A) fenestrated endothelium
(B) discontinuous endothelium
(C) continuous endothelium
(D) columnar epithelium

21. Nonencapsulated lymphoid organs are all except-
(A) payers patches
(B) vermiform appendix
(C) lymph node
(D) palatine tonsil

22. Organ having only efferent lymphatics is-
(A) lymph node
(B) spleen
(C) thymus
(D) tonsil

23. Thymus develops from-
(A) endoderm
(B) endoderm & mesoderm
(C) mesoderm & ectoderm
(D) endoderm, mesoderm & ectoderm

24. Thymus develops from –
(A) III branchial cleft
(B) III branchial pouch
(C) IV branchial pouch
(D) all of the above

25. Lymphocytes in the thymus are of-
(A) endodermal in origin
(B) mesodermal in origin
(C) ectodermal in origin
(D) A & B both

26. True about thymus is-
(A) lobulated lymphoid organ
(B) dark stained cortex and light stained medulla
(C) Hassall's corpuscles in medulla
(D) all of the above

27. Cells present in cortex of thymus are all except-
(A) thymocytes
(B) macrophages
(C) epithelial reticular cells
(D) B lymphocytes

28. Thymic hormones are secreted by-
(A) T lymphocytes
(B) macrophages
(C) epithelial reticular cells
(D) B lymphocytes

29. Hormones secreted from thymus are -
(A) thymulin
(B) thymosin
(C) thymopoietin
(D) all of the above

30. Lymph node is identified by presence of-
(A) sub capsular sinus
(B) lymphatic nodules in cortex
(C) capsule
(D) all of the above

31. Lymphatic nodules are absent in-
(A) lymph node
(B) spleen
(C) thymus
(D) tonsil

32. Primary lymphatic nodule is-
(A) nodule with germinal centre
(B) nodule without germinal centre
(C) nodule with eccentric arteriole
(D) nodules in red pulp

33. Secondary lymphatic nodule is-
(A) nodule with germinal centre
(B) nodule without germinal centre
(C) nodule with eccentric arteriole
(D) nodules in red pulp

34. T lymphocytes in lymph node are seen in –
(A) paracortex
(B) medulla
(C) hilum
(D) capsule

35. Largest lymphoid organ of the body is-
(A) thymus
(B) spleen
(C) tonsil
(D) hilar lymph nodes

36. Medulla of lymph node has-
(A) B lymphocytes
(B) plasma cells
(C) macrophages
(D) all of the above

37. Graveyard of RBC's is the name given to-
(A) thymus
(B) spleen
(C) lymph nodes
(D) all of the above

38. Spleen is-
(A) haemopoietic function
(B) reservoir of blood
(C) destruction of RBC's
(D) all of the above

39. Identification of spleen is done by-
(A) thick capsule & absence of sub capsular sinus
(B) lymph nodule with arteriole in it
(C) red pulp having sinusoids & splenic cords
(D) all of the above

40. Penicillar arterioles are seen in-
(A) lymph node
(B) spleen
(C) kidney
(D) all of the above

41. Stave cells are –
(A) seen in splenic venous sinuses
(B) spindle shaped endothelial cells
(C) present at gaps of basement membrane
(D) all of the above

42. Typical features of palatine tonsil is-
(A) crypts lined by stratified squamous epithelium
(B) sub epithelial lymphatic nodule
(C) mucous glands
(D) all of the above

43. Cords of Bilroth are seen in–
(A) subscapular sinus in lymph node
(B) blood thymus barrier
(C) red pulp of spleen
(D) white pulp of spleen

44. Hassall's corpuscles are –
(A) basophilic bodies
(B) eosiniphilic bodies
(C) both A & B
(D) none of the above

Answer Sheet

1 (D)	2 (B)	3 (B)	4 (A)	5 (C)	6 (B)	7 (B)	8 (A)	9 (A)	10 (A)
11 (D)	12 (D)	13 (C)	14 (B)	15 (D)	16 (B)	17 (B)	18 (C)	19 (D)	20 (B)
21 (C)	22 (C)	23 (B)	24 (B)	25 (B)	26 (D)	27 (D)	28 (A)	29 (D)	30 (D)
31 (C)	32 (B)	33 (A)	34 (A)	35 (B)	36 (D)	37 (B)	38 (D)	39 (D)	40 (B)
41 (D)	42 (D)	43 (C)	44 (B)						

Chapter 5

Muscular Tissue

1. Which of the following muscle has good regenerative capacity?
(A) Red skeletal muscle
(B) White skeletal muscle
(C) cardiac muscle
(D) smooth muscle

2. The cardiac muscle can be identified by the presence of-
(A) Intercalated disc
(B) Flat peripheral nuclei
(C) Caveolae
(D) Triads

3. In the skeletal muscle sarcosomes are–
(A) ribosomes
(B) mitochondria
(C) endoplasmic retinaculum
(D) all of the above

4. Skeletal muscle has –
(A) large central nucleus
(B) multiple central nuclei
(C) multiple flat peripheral nuclei
(D) multiple raised peripheral nuclei

5. The red skeletal muscle fibre is characterised by the presence of -
(A) high content of myoglobin
(B) many mitochondria
(C) rich blood supply
(D) all of the above

6. Purkinje fibres of heart are made of-
(A) autonomic nervous plexus
(B) collagen fibres
(C) modified cardiac muscle fibres
(D) modified nerve fibres

7. Loose connective tissue supporting the muscle fibre is called-
(A) perimysium
(B) endomysium
(C) epimysium
(D) endoneurium

8. Skeletal muscle shows-
(A) no branching
(B) multiple flat peripheral nucleus
(C) fibres show cross striations
(D) all of the above

9. Z line intersects –
(A) Dark band
(B) Light band
(C) Both A & B
(D) None of the above

10. Sarcomere is a space between –
(A) two A bands
(B) two I bands
(C) two Z lines
(D) all of the above

11. Thick filament is composed of-
(A) myosin
(B) actin
(C) troponin
(D) tropomyosin

12. Thin filament is composed of all except-
(A) myosin
(B) actin
(C) troponin
(D) tropomyosin

13. Thick filaments occupy –
(A) A band
(B) I band
(C) Z line
(D) M line

14. During contraction of skeletal muscle–
(A) shortening of thick filaments
(B) shortening of thin filament
(C) shortening of thick & thin filaments both
(D) none of the above

15. During contraction of skeletal muscle–
(A) shortening of A band
(B) lengthening of A band
(C) A band remains constant in width
(D) none of the above

16. During contraction of skeletal muscle–
(A) I band becomes narrow
(B) I band becomes expands
(C) I band remains constant in width
(D) none of the above

17. During contraction of skeletal muscle–
(A) H band becomes narrow
(B) H band becomes expands
(C) H band remains constant in width
(D) none of the above

18. During contraction of skeletal muscle–
(A) A band remains constant
(B) I & H band become narrow
(C) Z lines are drawn closer
(D) all of the above

19. System of T tubules for muscular contraction is at-
(A) A band
(B) I band
(C) junction between A & I bands
(D) at Z line

20. Ion necessary and released during muscular contraction is-
(A) Calcium
(B) Magnesium
(C) Iron
(D) Phosphorus

21. True about red muscle or aerobic type I muscle fibres-
(A) high myoglobin
(B) high cytochrome
(C) numerous mitochondria
(D) all of the above

22. True about red muscle or aerobic type I muscle fibres-
(A) rich blood supply
(B) postural muscles
(C) slow and continuous contractions
(D) all of the above

23. Succinate dehydrogenase myosin ATPase-
(A) present in red muscle
(B) present in white muscle
(C) present in both red & white muscle
(D) none of the above

24. Extra ocular muscles are-
(A) type I muscle fibres
(B) type II muscle fibres
(C) both type I & type II
(D) none of the above

25. Type II muscle fibres are-
(A) white muscle fibres
(B) anaerobic type
(C) Succinate dehydrogenase myosin ATPase (-)
(D) all of the above

26. Muscle spindles are-
(A) encapsulated stretch receptors
(B) made up of sensory nerve endings & intrafusal muscle fibres
(C) proprioceptive functions
(D) all of the above

27. Smooth muscle is seen in –
(A) arrector pili muscle
(B) Ciliary muscle
(C) sphincter pupillae
(D) all of the above

28. Smooth muscle is having-
(A) spindle shaped cells
(B) elongated central single nucleus
(C) striations are absent
(D) all of the above

29. True statement is-
(A) smooth muscle has striations
(B) skeletal muscle have branching
(C) cardiac muscle have branching
(D) all are true

30. Cardiac muscle shows-
(A) cross striations
(B) involuntary
(C) branching
(D) all of the above

31. Cardiac muscle shows-
(A) dark & light bands
(B) intercalated disc & branching
(C) central nuclei
(D) all of the above

32. Conducting system of heart is made up of-
(A) nerve fibres
(B) modified cardiac muscle fibres
(C) smooth muscle fibres
(D) none of the above

33. In smooth muscle T tubules are present at-
(A) at AI junction
(B) at Z line
(C) not present
(D) all of the above

34. In cardiac muscle T tubules are present at-
(A) at AI junction
(B) at Z line
(C) not present
(D) all of the above

35. In skeletal muscle T tubules are present at-
(A) at AI junction
(B) at Z line
(C) not present
(D) all of the above

36. The caveolae are seen in-
(A) cardiac muscle
(B) smooth muscle
(C) skeletal muscle
(D) all of the above

37. Regenerative capacity is minimal in-
(A) smooth muscle
(B) skeletal muscle
(C) cardiac muscle
(D) all of the above

38. Sarcoplasmic retinaculum forms triads in-
(A) smooth muscle
(B) skeletal muscle
(C) cardiac muscle
(D) all of the above

39. Sarcoplasmic retinaculum forms diads in-
(A) smooth muscle
(B) skeletal muscle
(C) cardiac muscle
(D) all of the above

40. Mitochondria in maximum number are seen in-
(A) smooth muscle
(B) skeletal muscle
(C) cardiac muscle
(D) none of the above

41. Mitochondria in least number are seen in-
(A) smooth muscle
(B) skeletal muscle
(C) cardiac muscle
(D) none of the above

42. Purkinje's fibres of myocardium are seen in-
(A) endocardium
(B) sub endocardium
(C) epicardium
(D) myocardium

43. Purkinje's fibres of myocardium are -
(A) rich in glycogen
(B) seen in sub endocardium
(C) larger than cardiac muscle fibres
(D) all of the above

44. Cardiac muscle fibre is about-
(A) 5 μm
(B) 10 μm
(C) 15 μm
(D) 25 μm

Answer Sheet

1 (D)	2 (A)	3 (B)	4 (C)	5 (D)	6 (C)	7 (B)	8 (D)	9 (B)	10 (C)
11 (A)	12 (A)	13 (A)	14 (D)	15 (C)	16 (A)	17 (A)	18 (D)	19 (C)	20 (A)
21 (D)	22 (D)	23 (A)	24 (B)	25 (D)	26 (D)	27 (D)	28 (D)	29 (C)	30 (D)
31 (D)	32 (B)	33 (C)	34 (B)	35 (A)	36 (B)	37 (C)	38 (B)	39 (C)	40 (C)
41 (A)	42 (B)	43 (D)	44 (C)						

Chapter 6

Nervous Tissue

1. Pseudo-unipolar neurons are found in the following ganglion-
(A) spinal
(B) spiral
(C) sympathetic
(D) parasympathetic

2. The connective tissue sheath around a nerve is called-
(A) endoneurium
(B) perineurium
(C) epineurium
(D) neurilemma

3. Section of sympathetic ganglion can be identified by the presence of-
(A) large pseudo-unipolar neuron
(B) small multipolar neurons
(C) bipolar neurons
(D) Well developed satellite cells

4. Betz cells are seen in-
(A) cerebellar cortex
(B) cerebellar nuclei
(C) sensory cortex of cerebrum
(D) motor cortex of cerebrum

5. Climbing fibres of cerebellum are-
(A) association fibres
(B) axons of purkinje cells
(C) efferent fibres
(D) afferent fibres

6. Total number of neurons in human being are-
(A) 1 million
(B) 5 million
(C) 10 million
(D) 100 million

7. Mesencephalic nucleus of trigeminal nerve has –
(A) unipolar neuron
(B) pseudo-unipolar neuron
(C) bipolar neuron
(D) multipolar neuron

8. Dorsal nerve root ganglion has –
(A) unipolar neuron
(B) pseudo-unipolar neuron
(C) bipolar neuron
(D) multipolar neuron

9. Spiral ganglion has –
(A) unipolar neuron
(B) pseudo-unipolar neuron
(C) bipolar neuron
(D) multipolar neuron

10. Autonomic parasympathetic ganglions has –
    (A) unipolar neuron
    (B) pseudo-unipolar neuron
    (C) bipolar neuron
    (D) multipolar neuron

11. Retina of the eye has –
    (A) unipolar neuron
    (B) pseudo-unipolar neuron
    (C) bipolar neuron
    (D) multipolar neuron

12. Cell bodies of neurons are located in-
    (A) grey matter of CNS
    (B) ganglion of PNS
    (C) both A & B
    (D) none of the above

13. Nissl bodies are aggregations of –
    (A) golgi bodies
    (B) smooth endoplasmic retinaculum
    (C) rough endoplasmic retinaculum
    (D) mitochondria

14. Nissl bodies are –
    (A) basophilic aggregations
    (B) seen in dendrites
    (C) modified rough endoplasmic retinaculum
    (D) all of the above

15. Nissl bodies are not seen in –
    (A) cell body
    (B) dendrites
    (C) axons
    (D) all of the above

16. Residual bodies are made up of-
    (A) golgi bodies
    (B) lysosomes
    (C) ribosomes
    (D) smooth endoplasmic retinaculum

17. Residual bodies are made up of-
    (A) melanin pigment
    (B) lipofuschin pigment
    (C) iron pigment
    (D) copper

18. True about the axon is-
    (A) uniform diameter
    (B) commonly referred as nerves
    (C) regeneration is possible if cell body is intact
    (D) all of the above

19. Axon hillock is having-
    (A) microtubules
    (B) microtubules & Nissl granules
    (C) microtubules but no Nissl granules
    (D) Nissl granules but no microtubules

20. Axons are mylinated by-
    (A) oligodendrocytes in CNS
    (B) Schwann cells in PNS
    (C) both A & B
    (D) none of the above

21. Chromatolysis is injury to axons and -
    (A) disintegration of lipofuschin
    (B) disintegration of dopamine
    (C) disintegration of Nissl granules
    (D) all of the above

22. Schmidt – Lantermann clefts are seen in-
    (A) within cell body
    (B) within dendrites
    (C) within myelin sheath
    (D) all of the above

23. Peripheral nerve is identified on microscopy by-
    (A) bundles of nerve fibres
    (B) perineurium around each bundle
    (C) darkly stained axons and lightly stained myelin
    (D) all of the above

24. Optic nerve is identified on microscopy by-
(A) bundles of myelinated nerve fibres
(B) Pia, arachnoid and duramater around each bundle
(C) central vessels of retina
(D) all of the above

25. Sympathetic ganglion is identified on microscopy by-
(A) small, scattered angular multipolar neurons of uniform size
(B) poorly defined satellite cells
(C) eccentrically placed nuclei in perikaryon
(D) all of the above

26. Well defined satellite cells are seen in–
(A) sympathetic ganglion
(B) motor ganglion (autonomic)
(C) sensory somatic ganglion
(D) all of the above

27. Dorsal nerve ganglion is identified on microscopy by-
(A) rounded pseudo-unipolar neurons of different size
(B) well defined satellite cells
(C) centrically placed nuclei in perikaryon
(D) all of the above

28. True about ependyma is-
(A) simple low columnar epithelium
(B) lacks basement membrane
(C) lines ventricles of brain & central canal of spinal cord
(D) all of the above

29. Neuroglia cells are-
(A) astrocytes
(B) oligodendrocytes
(C) microglial cells
(D) all of the above

30. All are ectodermal in origin except-
(A) astrocytes
(B) oligodendrocytes
(C) microglial cells
(D) all of the above

31. Microglial cells are derived from-
(A) ectoderm
(B) mesoderm
(C) endoderm
(D) all of the above

32. Most common cell in cerebral hemisphere is-
(A) pyramidal cell
(B) stellate cell
(C) horizontal cell of Cajal
(D) cells of Martinotti

33. Most superficial layer of cerebral cortex is-
(A) molecular layer
(B) external granular layer
(C) multiform layer
(D) internal pyramidal layer

34. Deepest layer of cerebral cortex is-
(A) molecular layer
(B) external granular layer
(C) multiform layer
(D) internal pyramidal layer

35. Cerebellum has three layers except-
(A) Purkinje cell layer
(B) granular layer
(C) multiform layer
(D) molecular layer

36. Smallest cell in the body are-
(A) purkinje cells
(B) pyramidal cells
(C) granular cells
(D) stellate cells

37. **Mossy fibres end into –**
(A) purkinje cells
(B) stellate cells
(C) granule cells
(D) none of the above

38. **Satellite cells in sensory ganglion are-**
(A) squamous cells
(B) cuboidal cells
(C) columnar cells
(D) all of the above

39. **Function of microglia is –**
(A) myelination
(B) phagocytosis
(C) secretion/absorption of CSF
(D) support & nourishment

40. **Function of oligodendrocytes is –**
(A) myelination
(B) phagocytosis
(C) secretion/absorption of CSF
(D) support & nourishment

41. **Function of astrocytes is –**
(A) myelination
(B) phagocytosis
(C) secretion/absorption of CSF
(D) support & nourishment

42. **Function of ependyma is –**
(A) myelination
(B) phagocytosis
(C) secretion/absorption of CSF
(D) support & nourishment

43. **Myelin sheath stains black with-**
(A) toluidine blue
(B) osmic acid
(C) silver stains
(D) India ink

44. **Nissl granules are stained with-**
(A) toluidine blue
(B) osmic acid
(C) silver stains
(D) India ink

45. **Aging pigment of nervous system is-**
(A) dopamine
(B) lipofuschin
(C) substantia nigra
(D) Nissl granules

Answer Sheet

1 (A)	2 (C)	3 (B)	4 (D)	5 (D)	6 (D)	7 (A)	8 (B)	9 (C)	10 (D)
11 (C)	12 (C)	13 (C)	14 (D)	15 (C)	16 (B)	17 (B)	18 (D)	19 (C)	20 (C)
21 (C)	22 (C)	23 (D)	24 (D)	25 (D)	26 (C)	27 (D)	28 (D)	29 (D)	30 (C)
31 (B)	32 (A)	33 (A)	34 (C)	35 (C)	36 (C)	37 (C)	38 (B)	39 (B)	40 (A)
41 (D)	42 (C)	43 (B)	44 (A)	45 (B)					

Chapter 7

Integumentary System - Skin

1. Thick skin is characterised by the presence of-
(A) Thick dermis
(B) Long interlocking epidermal ridges with dermal papillae
(C) Thick basement membrane
(D) All of the above

2. Thin skin is characterised by the presence of-
(A) Thin epidermis
(B) Hair follicle
(C) Sebaceous gland
(D) All of the above

3. Which of the following cells of epidermis is part of the immune system?
(A) Keratinocyte
(B) Melanocyte
(C) Langerhans cell
(D) Merkel's cell

4. Surface area of skin is about-
(A) 12 square feet
(B) 18 square feet
(C) 24 square feet
(D) 36 square feet

5. Heaviest organ of the body is-
(A) liver
(B) skin
(C) uterus
(D) kidney

6. Largest sense organ of the body is-
(A) brain
(B) skin
(C) bone
(D) olfactory system

7. Skin plays role in all of the following –
(A) excretion
(B) blood pressure regulation
(C) temperature regulation
(D) all of the above

8. Glabrous skin or thick skin has-
(A) very thick stratum corneum
(B) thick epidermis
(C) non hairy
(D) all are true

9. True about epidermis is all except-
(A) free nerve endings in basal layer
(B) ectodermal in origin
(C) is avascular
(D) renewed every 45-60days

10. Deepest layer of epidermis is-
(A) stratum basale
(B) stratum spongiosum
(C) stratum lucidum
(D) stratum corneum

11. True about stratum basale of epidermis is all except-
(A) single layer of cuboidal layer on basement membrane
(B) stratified squamous epithelium
(C) mitotic figures are seen
(D) deepest layer

12. Melanocytes are seen in-
(A) stratum basale of epidermis
(B) derived from neural crest
(C) round in shape and appear as clear cell in H%E
(D) all of the above

13. Keratinocytes in epidermis is -
(A) most common type of cells
(B) produces scleroprotiens - keratin
(C) fibrillar proteins / tonofibrils
(D) all of the above

14. Flattened eosinophilic dead cells are seen in-
(A) stratum basale
(B) stratum granulosum
(C) stratum spongiosum
(D) stratum lucidum

15. The cutaneous receptor concerned with pressure is-
(A) Pacinian corpuscle
(B) Meissner's corpuscle
(C) Free nerve ending
(D) Peritrichial nerve ending

16. The secretory tubules of sweat gland can be differentiated from the duct part by-
(A) Simple cuboidal epithelial lining
(B) stratified cuboidal epithelial lining
(C) smaller diameter of the tubule
(D) darker staining reaction with routine stains

17. Melanosomes are –
(A) melanocytes filled vesicles
(B) tyrosine filled vesicles
(C) melanophore filled vesicles
(D) all of the above

18. Absence of tyrosinase activity is seen in-
(A) psoriasis
(B) albinism
(C) sebhorrea dermatitis
(D) acne vulgaris

19. Langerhans cells are seen in-
(A) stratum spongiosum
(B) stratum granulosum
(C) stratum lucidum
(D) stratum basale

20. Bisbeck granules are seen in –
(A) melanocytes
(B) keratinocytes
(C) Langerhans cells
(D) merkel's cell

21. Langerhans cells are seen in all except-
(A) oral mucosa
(B) anal mucosa
(C) vagina
(D) thymus

22. True about Langerhans cells is all except -
(A) mesodermal in origin
(B) ectodermal in origin
(C) antigen presenting cell
(D) part of mononuclear phagocytic system

23. True about Langerhans cells is -
(A) Bisbeck granules
(B) absence of tonofilaments
(C) absence of desmosomes
(D) all of the above

24. Normally keratinization of skin takes about –
(A) 100-120 days
(B) 75-100 days
(C) 40-60 days
(D) 07-30days

25. In psoriasis keratinization of skin takes about –
(A) within a week
(B) 15-30 days
(C) 30-60 days
(D) 60-90days

26. Leather in commercial use is derived from-
(A) epidermis of skin
(B) dermis of skin
(C) A & B both
(D) none of the above

27. Dermis of skin corresponds to-
(A) mucosa of mucous membrane
(B) lamina propria of mucous membrane
(C) sub mucosa of mucous membrane
(D) adventitia of mucous membrane

28. Dermis contain smooth muscles in-
(A) face
(B) scrotum
(C) penis
(D) nipple

29. Secretions of sebaceous glands is controlled by –
(A) testosterone
(B) adrenal androgens
(C) oestrogens
(D) all of the above

30. Duct of sebaceous glands open into hair follicle except-
(A) glans penis
(B) clitoris
(C) lips
(D) all of the above

31. Sebaceous gland is classified as-
(A) merocrine
(B) apocrine
(C) Holocrine
(D) all of the above

32. Sweat glands are absent in –
(A) glans penis
(B) inner surface of prepuce
(C) margin of lips
(D) all of the above

33. Duct of sweat glands is lined with-
(A) stratified squamous epithelium
(B) stratified cuboidal epithelium
(C) stratified columnar epithelium
(D) simple cuboidal epithelium

34. Sweat glands are –
(A) merocrine
(B) apocrine
(C) A & B both
(D) Holocrine

35. Secretory tubules of sweat glands are made up of-
(A) simple columnar epithelium
(B) simple cuboidal epithelium
(C) stratified cuboidal epithelium
(D) stratified columnar epithelium

36. True about merocrine sweat gland is-
(A) present in dermis
(B) wide distribution in body
(C) open on epidermal surface
(D) all of the above

37. True about apocrine sweat gland is-
(A) present in hypodermis
(B) seen in axilla, external genitalia, anus and areola of nipple
(C) open on the hair follicle
(D) all of the above

38. Following are modified sweat gland except -
(A) mammary gland
(B) moll's gland of eyelid
(C) Ceruminious glands of external auditory meatus
(D) glands of Zies of eyelid

39. Following are modified sebaceous glands -
(A) tarsal gland of eyelid
(B) moll's gland of eyelid
(C) glands of Zies of eyelid
(D) A & C both

40. Hair are not present on-
(A) proximal phalanx
(B) middle phalanx
(C) distal phalanx
(D) all of the above

41. Terminal hair are seen in-
(A) scalp
(B) axilla
(C) pubic region
(D) all of the above

42. Non encapsulated receptor is-
(A) missener's corpuscle
(B) Pacinian corpuscle
(C) merkel's corpuscle
(D) ruffini's corpuscle

43. Receptor for two point tactile discrimination is -
(A) missener's corpuscle
(B) Pacinian corpuscle
(C) merkel's corpuscle
(D) ruffini's corpuscle

44. Receptor for pressure and vibration is-
(A) missener's corpuscle
(B) Pacinian corpuscle
(C) merkel's corpuscle
(D) ruffini's corpuscle

45. Receptor for stretch is-
(A) missener's corpuscle
(B) Pacinian corpuscle
(C) merkel's corpuscle
(D) ruffini's corpuscle

46. Receptor for pain and touch is-
(A) missener's corpuscle
(B) Pacinian corpuscle
(C) free nerve endings
(D) ruffini's corpuscle

47. Receptor having sliced onion appearance is-
(A) missener's corpuscle
(B) Pacinian corpuscle
(C) merkel's corpuscle
(D) ruffini's corpuscle

48. Glomera in the skin -
(A) controls colour of skin
(B) temperature regulation
(C) blood pressure regulation
(D) all of the above

Answer Sheet

1 (B)	2 (D)	3 (C)	4 (B)	5 (B)	6 (B)	7 (D)	8 (D)	9 (D)	10 (A)
11 (B)	12 (D)	13 (D)	14 (D)	15 (A)	16 (A)	17 (B)	18 (B)	19 (A)	20 (C)
21 (B)	22 (B)	23 (D)	24 (C)	25 (A)	26 (B)	27 (B)	28 (A)	29 (D)	30 (D)
31 (C)	32 (D)	33 (B)	34 (C)	35 (B)	36 (D)	37 (D)	38 (D)	39 (D)	40 (C)
41 (D)	42 (C)	43 (A)	44 (B)	45 (D)	46 (C)	47 (B)	48 (C)		

Chapter 8

Digestive System

1. Serous glands can be identified by the presence of serous acinus with-
   (A) Small lumen
   (B) Large lumen
   (C) Flat peripheral nuclei
   (D) Mucigen droplets

2. When there is a complete loss of cytoplasm resulting in death of the secretory cell during the process of secretion, the gland is said to be-
   (A) Merocrine
   (B) Apocrine
   (C) Holocrine
   (D) Cytocrine

3. Immunoglobin A is found in the secretion of which of the following?
   (A) Sublingual salivary glands
   (B) Parotid salivary glands
   (C) Submandibular salivary glands
   (D) Palatine glands

4. The isotonic primary saliva is converted into hypotonic saliva by secreting and absorbing certain ions by the-
   (A) Excretory duct
   (B) Secretory acini
   (C) Interlobular duct
   (D) Striated duct

5. The percentage of total volume of saliva secreted by submandibular gland is-
   (A) 70
   (B) 40
   (C) 25
   (D) 5

6. Cytocrine gland is –
   (A) sebaceous gland
   (B) testes
   (C) mammary gland
   (D) tarsal gland

7. Apocrine gland is –
   (A) sebaceous gland
   (B) testes
   (C) mammary gland
   (D) tarsal gland

8. Apocrine gland is –
   (A) sweat gland in genitalia
   (B) mammary gland
   (C) sweat glands in axilla
   (D) all of the above

9. Holocrine gland is –
(A) sebaceous gland
(B) testes
(C) mammary gland
(D) sweat gland

10. Holocrine gland is –
(A) salivary gland
(B) testes
(C) mammary gland
(D) tarsal gland

11. Serous gland is –
(A) parotid gland
(B) sublingual
(C) mammary gland
(D) submandibular gland

12. Mucous gland is –
(A) parotid gland
(B) sublingual
(C) mammary gland
(D) submandibular gland

13. Mixed gland is –
(A) parotid gland
(B) sublingual
(C) mammary gland
(D) submandibular gland

14. Zymogen granules in the apical part are seen in-
(A) mucous gland
(B) serous gland
(C) sebaceous gland
(D) all of the above

15. Goblet cell is an example of-
(A) Holocrine gland
(B) merocrine gland
(C) unicellular gland
(D) paracrine gland

16. Serous demilunes of Giannuzzi are seen in-
(A) parotid gland
(B) sublingual gland
(C) submandibular gland
(D) all of the above

17. The percentage of total volume of saliva secreted by submandibular gland is-
(A) 70
(B) 40
(C) 25
(D) 5

18. Dentine of the tooth is formed by-
(A) Ameloblast
(B) Odontoblast
(C) Cementoblast
(D) Fibroblast

19. Odontoblasts originate from-
(A) ectoderm
(B) mesoderm
(C) endoderm
(D) all of the above

20. Formation of dentine takes place during-
(A) foetal period
(B) childhood
(C) throughout life
(D) none of the above

21. Hardest substance of the body is-
(A) dentine
(B) enamel
(C) bone
(D) none of the above

22. Enamel is formed by-
(A) Ameloblast
(B) Odontoblast
(C) Cementoblast
(D) Fibroblast

23. Ameloblasts originate from-
(A) ectoderm
(B) mesoderm
(C) endoderm
(D) all of the above

24. True about cementoblasts of tooth is-
(A) secret cement throughout life
(B) become mature into cementocytes
(C) cementocytes remain in lacuna
(D) all of the above

25. Von Ebner's glands are seen in-
(A) tongue
(B) duodenum
(C) colon
(D) rectum

26. Tongue papilla covered with keratin is-
(A) filiform
(B) fungiform
(C) circumvallate
(D) foliate

27. Taste buds are absent in-
(A) filiform papilla
(B) fungiform papilla
(C) circumvallate papilla
(D) foliate papilla

28. Most common papilla of the tongue is–
(A) filiform papilla
(B) fungiform papilla
(C) circumvallate papilla
(D) foliate papilla

29. Taste buds not having any gland is-
(A) filiform papilla
(B) fungiform papilla
(C) circumvallate papilla
(D) foliate papilla

30. Circumvallate papilla is characterised by the presence of the following except-
(A) Circular furrow
(B) Taste buds on the lateral wall
(C) Simple columnar epithelium
(D) Von Ebner's glands

31. In addition to tongue taste buds are also present at-
(A) epiglottis
(B) soft palate
(C) oropharynx
(D) all of the above

32. Cells present in taste buds are-
(A) gustatory cells type II
(B) sustentacular cells
(C) basal cells
(D) all of the above

33. Sweet taste sensations are perceived from-
(A) tip of the tongue
(B) margin of the tongue in anterior 2/3
(C) dorsum of the tongue
(D) posterior part of the tongue

34. Salt taste sensations are perceived from-
(A) tip of the tongue
(B) margin of the tongue in anterior 2/3
(C) dorsum of the tongue
(D) posterior part of the tongue

35. Sour taste sensations are perceived from-
(A) tip of the tongue
(B) margin of the tongue in anterior 2/3
(C) central portion of the tongue
(D) posterior part of the tongue

36. Bitter taste sensations are perceived from-
(A) tip of the tongue
(B) margin of the tongue in anterior 2/3
(C) dorsum of the tongue
(D) posterior part of the tongue

37. Meissner's plexus is present in which layer of GIT?
(A) Lamina propria
(B) Submucosa
(C) Muscularis externa
(D) Serosa

38. Auerbach's nerve plexus is present in which layer of GIT?
(A) Lamina propria
(B) Submucosa
(C) Muscularis externa
(D) Serosa

39. Circular muscle layer in muscularis mucosa is absent in-
(A) oesophagus
(B) stomach
(C) small intestine
(D) colon

40. Muscularis externa of oesophagus in upper 1/3 shows-
(A) only skeletal muscle
(B) skeletal & smooth muscle both
(C) only smooth muscle
(D) none of the above

41. Muscularis externa of oesophagus in middle 1/3 shows-
(A) only skeletal muscle
(B) skeletal & smooth muscle both
(C) only smooth muscle
(D) none of the above

42. Muscularis externa of oesophagus in lower 1/3 shows-
(A) only skeletal muscle
(B) skeletal & smooth muscle both
(C) only smooth muscle
(D) none of the above

43. True about oesophagus is-
(A) no glands
(B) mucous glands in mucosa
(C) mucous glands in submucosa
(D) serous glands in submucosa

44. Glands of the stomach opens in-
(A) apex of the gastric pits
(B) middle of the gastric pits
(C) base of the gastric pits
(D) all of the above

45. Which of the following structure is not lined by stratified squamous epithelium?
(A) Oral cavity
(B) Oesophagus
(C) Stomach
(D) Anal canal

46. Stomach is lined with-
(A) simple columnar epithelium
(B) simple columnar ciliated epithelium
(C) pseudostratified columnar epithelium
(D) pseudostratified columnar ciliated epithelium

47. Fundic part of stomach shows-
(A) shallow gastric pits
(B) fundic glands in lamina propria
(C) chief & parietal/oxyntic cells
(D) all of the above

48. Pyloric part of stomach shows-
(A) deep gastric pits
(B) pyloric glands in lamina propria
(C) circular muscle thickening
(D) all of the above

49. Oesophageal-cardiac junction is having -
(A) stratified squamous epithelium
(B) simple columnar epithelium
(C) glands in lamina propria
(D) all of the above

50. Mucous neck cells are seen in-
(A) cardiac end of stomach
(B) body of stomach
(C) pyloric end of stomach
(D) all of the above

51. To facilitate absorption, the luminal surface area of small intestine is increased manifold due to the presence of-
(A) Plica circularis
(B) Intestinal villi
(C) Microvilli
(D) All of the above

52. Valves of Kerckring are –
(A) permanent folds of mucosa & submucosa
(B) seen in small intestine
(C) best developed in jejunum
(D) all of the above

53. Typical features of duodenum are-
(A) leaf like villi
(B) Brunner's glands in submucosa
(C) crypts of Lieberkuhn
(D) all of the above

54. Finger like villi are typical feature of-
(A) duodenum
(B) jejunum
(C) ileum
(D) colon

55. Peyer's patches are seen in-
(A) duodenum
(B) jejunum
(C) ileum
(D) appendix

56. Paneth cells are present in-
(A) Rectum
(B) Colon
(C) Small intestine
(D) Stomach

57. M cells are seen in-
(A) stomach
(B) ileum
(C) appendix
(D) anal canal

58. Intestinal villi are absent in-
(A) duodenum
(B) jejunum
(C) ileum
(D) sigmoid colon

59. Typical features of appendix is-
(A) lymphoid follicles in lamina propria
(B) disrupted muscularis mucosa
(C) no villi
(D) all of the above

60. Appendices epiploicae are seen in-
(A) appendix
(B) caecum
(C) rectum
(D) upper part of anal canal

61. Taeniae coli are absent in-
(A) caecum
(B) colon
(C) sigmoid colon
(D) rectum

62. Type of epithelium in anal canal is-
(A) stratified squamous
(B) stratified columnar
(C) stratified cuboidal
(D) all of the above

63. Type of epithelium in anal canal above the anal valves is-
(A) stratified squamous
(B) stratified columnar
(C) both A & B
(D) none of the above

64. Type of epithelium in anal canal below the anal valves is-
(A) stratified squamous
(B) stratified columnar
(C) both A & B
(D) none of the above

65. Typical features of anal canal are-
(A) rich venous plexus in submucosa
(B) no villi and no crypts of Lieberkuhn
(C) stratified squamous epithelium & no muscularis mucosa
(D) all of the above

66. The percentage of saliva secreted by submandibular gland is-
(A) 70
(B) 30
(C) 20
(D) 10

67. Percentage of saliva secreted by parotid gland –
(A) 5
(B) 20
(C) 30
(D) 70

68. Opening of main duct of salivary gland into oral cavity is lined by –
(A) stratified squamous epithelium
(B) stratified columnar epithelium
(C) stratified cuboidal epithelium
(D) all of the above

69. Striated duct(intra lobular) of salivary gland is lined by –
(A) stratified squamous epithelium
(B) stratified columnar epithelium
(C) stratified cuboidal epithelium
(D) all of the above

70. Inter lobular (excretory) duct of salivary gland is lined by –
(A) stratified squamous epithelium
(B) stratified columnar epithelium
(C) stratified cuboidal epithelium
(D) all of the above

71. All are true except-
(A) Parotid gland-serous
(B) submandibular gland-mucous
(C) sublingual gland- mucous
(D) submandibular – mixed

72. Serous demilunes are seen in-
(A) parotid & sublingual gland
(B) parotid & submandibular gland
(C) submandibular & sublingual gland
(D) parotid, submandibular & sublingual glands

73. Glisson's capsule is seen in-
(A) kidney
(B) adrenal
(C) liver
(D) gallbladder

74. True about Kupffer's cells is-
(A) part of mononuclear-macrophage system
(B) endothelia phagocytic cell
(C) seen in liver
(D) all of the above

75. **Portal tract or triad classically have all except-**
(A) portal vein
(B) bile duct
(C) hepatic vein
(D) hepatic artery

76. **Which of the following statements is not true about the striated ducts of salivary glands-**
(A) Are involved in ion transport
(B) Show basal infoldings of plasma membrane
(C) Bear microvilli on their free surface
(D) Are intralobular in position

77. **Bile canaliculus is lined by-**
(A) Endothelium
(B) Plasma membrane
(C) Cuboidal epithelium
(D) None of the above

78. **Secretion of glucagon in the islet of Langerhans is from-**
(A) Alpha
(B) Beta
(C) Delta
(D) None of the above

79. **Secretion of insulin in the islet of Langerhans is from-**
(A) Alpha
(B) Beta
(C) Delta
(D) None of the above

80. **Secretion of somatostatin in the islet of Langerhans is from-**
(A) Alpha
(B) Beta
(C) Delta
(D) None of the above

81. **Centroacinar cell is seen in-**
(A) parotid
(B) pancreas
(C) liver
(D) spleen

82. **Centroacinar cells of pancreas are of -**
(A) simple squamous type
(B) cuboidal type
(C) columnar type
(D) none of the above

83. **Ducts of pancreas are lined by-**
(A) simple columnar epithelium
(B) simple cuboidal epithelium
(C) stratified cuboidal epithelium
(D) stratified columnar epithelium

84. **True about beta cells of pancreas is-**
(A) small cell with basophilic granules
(B) large cell with acidophilic granules
(C) large cell with acidophilic granules
(D) small cell with basophilic granules

85. **True about alfa cells of pancreas is-**
(A) small cell with basophilic granules
(B) large cell with acidophilic granules
(C) large cell with basophilic granules
(D) small cell with acidophilic granules

86. **Cells seen in pancreas are-**
(A) alfa cells
(B) alfA & Beta cells
(C) alfa, beta & delta cells
(D) alfa, beta, delta & F-cells

87. **Typical features of gall bladder are-**
(A) lined by columnar epithelium with brush border
(B) muscularis mucosa & submucosa are absent
(C) fibromuscular layer
(D) all of the above

Answer Sheet

1. (A)	2 (C)	3 (B)	4 (D)	5 (A)	6 (B)	7 (C)	8 (D)	9 (A)	10 (D)
11 (A)	12 (B)	13 (D)	14 (B)	15 (C)	16 (C)	17 (C)	18 (B)	19. (B)	20 (C)
21 (B)	22 (A)	23 (A)	24 (D)	25 (A)	26 (A)	27 (A)	28 (A)	29 (A)	30 (C)
31 (D)	32 (D)	33 (A)	34 (B)	35 (C)	36 (D)	37 (B)	38 (C)	39 (A)	40 (A)
41 (B)	42 (C)	43 (C)	44 (C)	45 (C)	46 (A)	47 (D)	48 (D)	49 (D)	50 (B)
51 (D)	52 (D)	53 (D)	54 (B)	55 (C)	56 (C)	57 (B)	58 (D)	59 (D)	60 (B)
61 (D)	62 (D)	63 (B)	64 (A)	65 (D)	66 (A)	67 (B)	68 (A)	69 (C)	70 (B)
71 (B)	72 (C)	73 (C)	74 (D)	75 (C)	76 (C)	77 (B)	78 (A)	79 (B)	80 (C)
81 (B)	82 (B)	83 (C)	84 (A)	85 (B)	86 (D)	87 (D)			

Chapter 9

Urinary System

1. Cortex of the kidney contains the following structures except -
(A) proximal convoluted tubule(PCT)
(B) distal convoluted tubule (DCT)
(C) renal corpuscle
(D) thin segment of loop of Henle

2. The PCT can be identified in histological section by the presence of-
(A) Acidophilic cytoplasm of the lining of cuboidal cells
(B) Basophilic cytoplasm of the lining of cuboidal cells
(C) Pale staining cytoplasm
(D) Large lumen

3. Duct of Bellini are found in-
(A) liver
(B) adrenal
(C) kidney
(D) none of the above

4. Columns of Bertin are –
(A) medullary rays
(B) renal columns
(C) renal corpuscles
(D) renal papilla

5. Macula densa is present in -
(A) PCT
(B) DCT
(C) Afferent arteriole
(D) Efferent arteriole

6. All of the following statements are true about juxtaglomerular cells except that they are-
(A) Modified smooth muscle cells
(B) Sensitive to concentration of sodium ions
(C) Responsible for production of renin
(D) Found in afferent arteriole

7. Aldosterone acts on which of the following parts of uriniferous tubule?
(A) Collecting duct
(B) Collecting tubule
(C) DCT
(D) PCT

8. Nephron is developed from-
(A) uretric bud
(B) metanephric blastema
(C) paramesonephric duct
(D) all of the above

9. Short loop of Henle are seen in-
(A) cortical nephrons
(B) juxtamedullary nephrons
(C) both A & B
(D) none of the above

10. Parietal layer of Bowman's capsule is made up of-
(A) simple squamous
(B) simple cuboidal
(C) cuboidal with brush border
(D) all of the above

11. True about podocytes is-
(A) cells of visceral layer of bowman's capsule
(B) have primary & secondary foot processes
(C) form filtration pores
(D) all of the above

12. In renal corpuscle mesangial cells are-
(A) specialised connective tissue cells
(B) stellate cells having contractile & phagocytic potential
(C) clear the glomerular infiltrate
(D) all of the above

13. Thin segment of loop of Henle is made up of-
(A) simple squamous epithelium
(B) forms bulk of the renal cortex
(C) brush border appearance
(D) all of the above

14. True statement about loop of Henle is -
(A) thin segment is lined by squamous epithelium
(B) thick segment is lined by cuboidal epithelium
(C) thin segment is permeable to water
(D) all of the above

15. True about DCT is –
(A) is lined by cuboidal epithelium
(B) maintains acid balance
(C) Is impermeable to water
(D) All of the above

16. Papillary ducts (duct of Bellini) in kidney are lined with-
(A) Simple squamous epithelium
(B) Cuboidal epithelium
(C) Columnar epithelium
(D) All of the above

17. Collecting tubules in kidney are lined with-
(A) Simple squamous epithelium
(B) Cuboidal epithelium
(C) Columnar epithelium
(D) All of the above

18. True about Juxtaglomerular cells is-
(A) Modified smooth cells
(B) Present in tunica media
(C) Internal elastic lamina disappears at the site
(D) All of the above

19. JG cells are -
(A) Chemoreceptors
(B) Mechanoreceptors
(C) Baroreceptors
(D) None of the above

20. Macula densa cells are specialised cells in –
(A) Wall of PCT
(B) Wall of DCT
(C) Wall of Afferent arteriole
(D) wall of Efferent arteriole

21. Macula densa cells are –
(A) present in the DCT
(B) sensitive to sodium ion
(C) are osmoreceptors
(D) all of the above

22. **Polkissen cells are –**
(A) Extra glomerular mesangial cell
(B) found at vascular pole
(C) involvement in erythropoietin production
(D) all of the above

23. **Renin enzyme is secreted by-**
(A) Polkissen cells
(B) macula densa cells
(C) Juxtaglomerular cells
(D) all of the above

24. **True about the ureter is-**
(A) star shaped lumen
(B) transitional epithelium
(C) outer circular & inner longitudinal layers in muscularis externa
(D) all of the above

25. **Lower one third of ureter has -**
(A) outer circular & inner longitudinal muscle
(B) outer longitudinal & inner circular muscle
(C) outer circular & inner longitudinal muscle & outermost circular
(D) outer circular & inner longitudinal muscle & outermost longitudinal

26. **Female urethra is lined with-**
(A) transitional epithelium
(B) stratified squamous epithelium
(C) stratified cuboidal epithelium
(D) all of the above

27. **Umbrella cells are seen in-**
(A) urinary bladder
(B) uterus
(C) fallopian tube
(D) ductus deferens

Answer Sheet

1 (D)	2 (A)	3 (C)	4 (B)	5 (B)	6 (D)	7 (C)	8 (B)	9 (A)	10 (A)
11 (D)	12 (D)	13 (D)	14 (D)	15 (D)	16 (C)	17 (B)	18 (D)	19 (B)	20 (B)
21 (D)	22 (D)	23 (C)	24 (D)	25 (D)	26 (B)	27 (A)			

Chapter 10

Respiratory System

1. Septal cells of the lung alveoli are involved in-
(A) Blood-air barrier
(B) Phagocytosis
(C) Production of surfactant
(D) Allergic reaction

2. Respiratory epithelium is mainly –
(A) ciliated columnar epithelium
(B) stratified columnar epithelium
(C) pseudostratified columnar epithelium
(D) simple columnar epithelium

3. Submucosa of respiratory tract have glands except-
(A) trachea
(B) principal bronchus
(C) larynx
(D) bronchioles

4. Yellow olfactory mucosa is seen at-
(A) roof of nasal cavity
(B) lateral wall of nose
(C) superior part of nasal septum
(D) all of the above

5. Olfactory mucosa is made up of-
(A) olfactory cells
(B) sustentacular cells
(C) basal cells
(D) all of the above

6. Bowman's glands are seen in-
(A) kidney
(B) lamina propria of respiratory epithelium of nose
(C) lamina propria of olfactory epithelium of nose
(D) submucosa of olfactory epithelium

7. Olfactory cells in olfactory mucosa are-
(A) pseudo unipolar cells
(B) bipolar cells
(C) multipolar cells
(D) all of the above

8. Respiratory mucosa is made up of-
(A) columnar ciliated cells
(B) goblet cells
(C) basal cells
(D) all of the above

9. Respiratory mucosa is made up of-
(A) columnar ciliated cells
(B) granule cells
(C) brush cells
(D) all of the above

10. Respiratory mucosa is –
(A) pink in colour
(B) yellow in colour
(C) white in colour
(D) none of the above

11. Immotile cilia syndrome is due to-
(A) absence of protein desmin
(B) absence of protein dynein
(C) absence of protein motilin
(D) absence of protein flagellin

12. Which one of the following is an example of elastic cartilage?
(A) Epiglottis
(B) Cricoid cartilage
(C) Arytenoid cartilage
(D) Thyroid cartilage

13. Bowman's glands are present in-
(A) Submucosa of duodenum
(B) Submucosa of oesophagus
(C) Olfactory mucosa
(D) Cortex of kidney

14. Bronchiole is characterised by-
(A) Presence of Clara cells
(B) Absence of glands
(C) Absence of cartilage
(D) All of the above

15. Which of the following is not lined by stratified squamous epithelium?
(A) Oropharynx
(B) Nasopharynx
(C) Vocal cord
(D) Lingual surface of epiglottis

16. Epithelial lining of oropharynx is –
(A) stratified ciliated columnar
(B) pseudostratified ciliated columnar
(C) stratified squamous
(D) none of the above

17. Epithelial lining of nasopharynx is –
(A) stratified ciliated columnar
(B) pseudostratified ciliated columnar
(C) stratified squamous
(D) none of the above

18. Epithelial lining of larynx is –
(A) stratified ciliated columnar
(B) pseudostratified ciliated columnar
(C) stratified squamous
(D) none of the above

19. Epithelial lining of vocal cords is –
(A) stratified ciliated columnar
(B) pseudostratified ciliated columnar
(C) stratified squamous
(D) none of the above

20. Epithelial lining of epiglottis is –
(A) stratified ciliated columnar
(B) pseudostratified ciliated columnar
(C) stratified squamous
(D) both B & C

21. Trachea shows-
(A) C shaped hyaline cartilage
(B) pseudostratified ciliated columnar epithelium
(C) mixed tracheal glands in submucosa
(D) all of the above

22. Epithelial lining of alveoli is –
(A) stratified ciliated columnar
(B) pseudostratified ciliated columnar
(C) simple squamous
(D) stratified squamous

23. Epithelial lining of alveolar duct is –
(A) stratified ciliated columnar
(B) pseudostratified ciliated cuboidal
(C) simple squamous
(D) stratified squamous

24. Dust cells are-
(A) alveolar macrophages
(B) part of mononuclear macrophage system
(C) contain inhaled carbon particles
(D) all of the above

25. Pulmonary surfactant is secreted by-
(A) type I pneumocytes
(B) type II pneumocytes
(C) Clara cells
(D) none of the above

26. True about type I pneumocytes is-
(A) squamous epithelial cells
(B) cover 97% of alveolar surface is cover
(C) form part of blood air barrier
(D) all of the above

27. True about type II pneumocytes is all except-
(A) cuboidal cells with microvilli
(B) cover 3% of alveolar surface is cover
(C) form part of blood air barrier
(D) secrete lipoprotein - surfactant

28. Vestibule of the nose is lined with-
(A) olfactory mucosa
(B) respiratory mucosa
(C) skin
(D) all of the above

29. In bronchiole goblet cells are replaced by-
(A) macrophage
(B) clara cell
(C) type I pneumocytes
(D) type II pneumocytes

30. Removal of surfactant is done by-
(A) macrophage
(B) clara cell
(C) type I pneumocytes
(D) type II pneumocytes.

Answer Sheet

1 (C)	2 (C)	3 (D)	4 (D)	5 (D)	6 (C)	7 (B)	8 (D)	9 (D)	10 (A)
11 (B)	12 (A)	13 (C)	14 (D)	15 (B)	16 (C)	17 (B)	18 (B)	19 (C)	20 (D)
21 (D)	22 (C)	23 (C)	24 (D)	25 (B)	26 (D)	27 (C)	28 (C)	29 (B)	30 (C)

Chapter 11

Blood Vessels

1. A large artery is characterised by the presence of-
   (A) A well developed internal elastic lamina
   (B) Elastic fibres in tunica media
   (C) Smooth muscle fibres in tunica adventitia
   (D) Mesothelial lining

2. Endothelial lining of blood vessels is of-
   (A) simple squamous epithelium
   (B) simple cuboidal epithelium
   (C) simple columnar epithelium
   (D) all of the above

3. Atherosclerosis in artery is due to-
   (A) Thickening of tunica intima
   (B) Accumulation of lipid in myointimal cells
   (C) Calcification of tunica media
   (D) All of the above

4. Medium-sized artery is characterised by the presence of-
   (A) A well developed internal elastic lamina
   (B) A well developed sub endothelial connective tissue
   (C) Elastic fibres in tunica media
   (D) Smooth muscle fibres in tunica adventitia

5. Medium sized arteries are all except-
   (A) radial artery
   (B) ulnar artery
   (C) carotid artery
   (D) facial artery

6. Exchange vessels are-
   (A) arterioles
   (B) capillaries
   (C) venules
   (D) all of the above

7. Well developed capillary network is seen in-
   (A) cardiac muscle
   (B) kidney
   (C) liver
   (D) all of the above

8. Pericytes are-
   (A) Modified endothelial cells
   (B) Phagocytic cells
   (C) Pluripotent cells found in association with capillaries
   (D) Found in tunica media of arterioles

9. Continuous capillaries are seen in all except-
(A) brain
(B) lung
(C) kidney
(D) muscle

10. Most common type of capillary is-
(A) continuous capillary
(B) fenestrated capillary
(C) sinusoidal capillary
(D) none of the above

11. Fenestrated capillaries are seen in all except-
(A) thyroid
(B) intestinal villi
(C) kidney
(D) muscle

12. Sinusoidal capillaries are seen in all except-
(A) spleen
(B) liver
(C) kidney
(D) bone marrow

13. Lumen of capillary is about-
(A) 3-7μm
(B) 7-9μm
(B) 11-15μm
(D) 18-25μm

14. Natriuretic hormone is secreted by-
(A) atrial myocardial fibres
(B) endothelial wall of elastic artery
(C) ventricular myocardial fibres
(D) all of the above

15. Glomera are seen in the skin at the-
(A) tips of fingers & toes
(B) tip of tongue & lips
(C) nose
(D) all of the above

16. Glomus is made up of-
(A) efferent artery, connecting vessel & afferent vein
(B) afferent artery, connecting vessel & afferent vein
(C) afferent artery, connecting vessel & efferent vein
(D) none of the above

17. Arteriovenous anastomoses is seen at-
(A) thyroid
(B) sympathetic ganglia
(C) erectile tissue of genitalia
(D) all of the above

18. Muscles are completely absent in the following veins except-
(A) dural venous sinuses
(B) retinal vein
(C) vertebral veins
(D) Cancellous bone

19. Valves are absent in the following veins -
(A) dural venous sinuses
(B) vena cava
(C) vertebral veins
(D) all of the above

20. Sinusoids are seen in –
(A) parathyroid gland
(B) carotid body
(C) adrenal cortex
(D) all of the above

21. Diapedesis is noted in-
(A) vein
(B) venules
(C) arteriole
(D) all of the above

22. Pinocytosis is observed in-
(A) continuous capillaries
(B) fenestrated capillaries
(C) sinusoidal capillaries
(D) all of the above

23. Coronary arteries are an example of -
(A) elastic artery
(B) muscular artery
(C) arterioles
(D) all of the above

24. Elastic arteries are all except-
(A) subclavian artery
(B) axillary artery
(C) carotid artery
(D) iliac artery

25. Large vein has –
(A) thick muscular wall as compared to narrow circular lumen
(B) well developed tunica adventitia with bundle of smooth muscle
(C) well developed tunica media with elastic fibres
(D) well developed tunica media with muscle fibres

26. An arteriole has –
(A) thick muscular wall as compared to narrow circular lumen
(B) well developed tunica adventitia with bundle of smooth muscle
(C) well developed tunica media with elastic fibres
(D) well developed tunica media with muscle fibres

27. Medium sized artery has –
(A) thick muscular wall as compared to narrow circular lumen
(B) well developed tunica adventitia with bundle of smooth muscle
(C) well developed tunica media with elastic fibres
(D) well developed tunica media with muscle fibres

28. Large artery has –
(A) thick muscular wall as compared to narrow circular lumen
(B) well developed tunica adventitia with bundle of smooth muscle
(C) well developed tunica media with elastic fibres
(D) well developed tunica media with muscle fibres

29. True statement is-
(A) precapillary sphincter is seen in meta-arteriole
(B) diameter of sinusoidal capillary is uniform
(C) capillary of endocrine glands are lined with continuous endothelium
(D) internal elastic lamina is well developed in arterioles

30. Capillary endothelial cells are involved in-
(A) Conversion of angiotensin I to angiotensin II
(B) Exchange of metabolites
(C) Diapedesis
(D) All of the above

Answer Sheet

1 **(B)**	2 **(A)**	3 **(D)**	4 **(A)**	5 **(C)**	6 **(B)**	7 **(D)**	8 **(C)**	9 **(C)**	10 **(A)**
11 **(D)**	12 **(C)**	13 **(B)**	14 **(A)**	15 **(D)**	16 **(C)**	17 **(D)**	18 **(C)**	19 **(D)**	20 **(D)**
21 **(B)**	22 **(A)**	23 **(B)**	24 **(C)**	25 **(B)**	26 **(A)**	27 **(D)**	28 **(C)**	29 **(A)**	30 **(D)**

Chapter 12

Endocrine Glands

1. Adenohypophysis is derived from-
(A) Neural ectoderm
(B) Oral ectoderm
(C) Mesoderm
(D) Endoderm

2. Adenohypophysis is derived from -
(A) Neural ectoderm
(B) Rathke's pouch
(C) Mesoderm
(D) Endoderm

3. Neurohypophysis is derived from -
(A) Neural ectoderm
(B) Rathke's pouch
(C) Mesoderm
(D) Endoderm

4. Pituicytes & unmylinated nerve fibres are seen in-
(A) anterior pituitary
(B) posterior pituitary
(C) pituitary stalk
(D) all of the above

5. Herring bodies are seen in-
(A) anterior pituitary
(B) posterior pituitary
(C) pituitary stalk
(D) all of the above

6. Herring bodies in neurohypophysis store-
(A) oxytocin hormone
(B) vasopressin hormone
(C) oxytocin & vasopressin both
(D) none of the above

7. Smallest chromophil cells in pituitary gland are-
(A) somatotrophs
(B) lactotrophs
(C) thyrotrophs
(D) corticotrophs

8. Largest chromophil cells in pituitary gland are-
(A) somatotrophs
(B) lactotrophs
(C) thyrotrophs
(D) corticotrophs

9. Pars intermedia in human is supposed to secret-
(A) MSH
(B) ACTH
(C) LPH
(D) all of the above

10. Paraventricular nuclei are associated with secretion of-
   (A) oxytocin
   (B) vasopressin
   (C) both A & B
   (D) none of the above

11. Supra optic nuclei are associated with secretion of-
   (A) oxytocin
   (B) vasopressin
   (C) both A & B
   (D) none of the above

12. Thyroid gland develops from-
   (A) thyroglossal duct
   (B) ultimobranchial body
   (C) both A & B
   (D) none of the above

13. Epithelial lining of thyroid follicle is-
   (A) simple squamous epithelium
   (B) simple cuboidal epithelium
   (C) simple columnar epithelium
   (D) all of the above

14. Epithelial lining of classical thyroid follicle is-
   (A) simple squamous epithelium
   (B) simple cuboidal epithelium
   (C) simple columnar epithelium
   (D) all of the above

15. Epithelial lining of active thyroid follicle is-
   (A) simple squamous epithelium
   (B) simple cuboidal epithelium
   (C) simple columnar epithelium
   (D) all of the above

16. Epithelial lining of resting thyroid follicle is-
   (A) simple squamous epithelium
   (B) simple cuboidal epithelium
   (C) simple columnar epithelium
   (D) all of the above

17. Only endocrine gland which stores its secretion is-
   (A) pituitary gland
   (B) thyroid gland
   (C) adrenal medulla
   (D) parathyroid gland

18. Most abundant hormone secreted from thyroid gland is-
   (A) T3
   (B) T4
   (C) TSH
   (D) all of the above

19. Most potent hormone secreted from thyroid gland is-
   (A) T3
   (B) T4
   (C) TSH
   (D) all of the above

20. True about calcitonin hormone is-
   (A) secreted from C-cells or parafollicular cells of thyroid
   (B) secreted in response to blood calcium level
   (C) antagonist of parathormone
   (D) all of the above

21. Androgens are secreted from-
   (A) zona reticulosa
   (B) zona fasciculata
   (C) zona glomerulosa
   (D) medulla

22. Adrenal gland develops from-
   (A) mesoderm
   (B) neural crest
   (C) mesoderm & neural crest both
   (D) none of the above

23. glucocorticoids are secreted from-
(A) zona reticulosa
(B) zona fasciculata
(C) zona glomerulosa
(D) medulla

24. Aldosterone is secreted from-
(A) zona reticulosa
(B) zona fasciculata
(C) zona glomerulosa
(D) medulla

25. Largest zone of adrenal cortex is-
(A) zona reticulosa
(B) zona fasciculata
(C) zona glomerulosa
(D) medulla

26. Adrenaline & noradrenaline are secreted from-
(A) zona reticulosa
(B) zona fasciculata
(C) zona glomerulosa
(D) adrenal medulla

27. Pars intermedia lies between-
(A) Hypophyseal cleft and pars nervosa
(B) Hypophyseal cleft and pars distalis
(C) Pars distalis and pars tuberalis
(D) Pars tuberalis and pars nervosa

28. Parathyroid gland controls blood level of-
(A) increases calcium & phosphate level
(B) increases calcium & decrease phosphate level
(C) decreases both calcium & phosphate level
(D) none of the above

29. Parathormone raises blood calcium by-
(A) stimulates osteoclasts
(B) DCT to increase reabsorption
(C) synthesis of calcitriol the active form of vit D
(D) all of the above

30. Parathormone is secreted by Chief cells of parathyroid which are–
(A) smaller & polygonal in shape
(B) vesicular nucleus
(C) pale staining granular cytoplasm
(D) all are true

31. The hormones involved in breast development and lactation are-
(A) FSH and LH
(B) GH and TSH
(C) Prolactin and oxytocin
(D) Vasopressin and aldosterone

32. Thyroid gland differs from other endocrine glands in-
(A) Having anastomosing cords of cells
(B) Having less vasculature
(C) Storing the secretion intracellular
(D) Storing the secretion extracellularly

33. Which of the following is not true about the parafollicular cells? They-
(A) Secrete calcitonin
(B) Are also called C or clear cells
(C) Contain secretory granules in the cytoplasm
(D) Are dependent on pituitary hormone for their secretion

34. True about zona glomerulosa of suprarenal gland is all except –
(A) outer most zone & forms 1/7th of the adrenal gland
(B) inverted U shaped arched clusters of columnar/polyhedral cells
(C) continuous capillaries are seen here
(D) cytoplasm is acidophilic cells with lipid droplets

35. Mineralocorticosteroids ie aldosterone maintains water and electrolyte balance by-
(A) reabsorption of sodium from DCT of kidneys
(B) striated ducts of sweat & salivary glands
(C) from gastric mucosa
(D) all of the above

36. True about zona fasciculata of suprarenal gland is –
(A) largest zone & 2/3rd of the adrenal gland
(B) columns of polyhedral cells secreting glucocorticoids
(C) fenestrated capillaries are seen here
(D) all of the above

37. Chromaffin cells are seen in –
(A) zona glomerulosa
(B) zona fasciculata
(C) adrenal medulla
(D) zona reticulosa

38. Secretory granules are seen in the –
(A) zona glomerulosa
(B) zona fasciculata
(C) adrenal medulla
(D) zona reticulosa

39. Third eye is name given to-
(A) pituitary
(B) pineal gland
(C) superior colliculus
(D) all of the above

40. Brain sand or corpora arenacea is seen in-
(A) pituitary
(B) pineal gland
(C) superior colliculus
(D) substantia nigra

41. Cells seen in Pineal gland –
(A) pinealocytes
(B) astroglial cells
(C) interstitial cells
(D) all of the above

42. Brain sand or corpora arenacea is made up of-
(A) basophilic bodies
(B) calcium & magnesium
(C) increases with age
(D) all of the above

43. Pinealocytes secrete –
(A) norepinephrine
(B) serotonin
(C) melatonin
(D) all of the above

Answer Sheet

1 **(B)**	2 **(B)**	3 **(A)**	4 **(B)**	5 **(B)**	6 **(C)**	7 **(C)**	8 **(D)**	9 **(D)**	10 **(A)**
11 **(B)**	12 **(C)**	13 **(D)**	14 **(B)**	15 **(C)**	16 **(A)**	17 **(B)**	18 **(B)**	19 **(A)**	20 **(D)**
21 **(A)**	22 **(C)**	23 **(B)**	24 **(C)**	25 **(B)**	26 **(D)**	27 **(A)**	28 **(B)**	29 **(D)**	30 **(D)**
31 **(C)**	32 **(D)**	33 **(D)**	34 **(C)**	35 **(D)**	36 **(D)**	37 **(C)**	38 **(C)**	39 **(B)**	40 **(B)**
41 **(D)**	42 **(D)**	43 **(D)**							